03

ᘓ

Handbook of Asthma
and Rhinitis

Handbook of Asthma and Rhinitis

Robert K. Bush, MD

Professor
Section of Allergy and Clinical Immunology
University of Wisconsin-Madison Medical School
Chief of Allergy
William S. Middleton Veteran Administration Hospital
Madison, Wisconsin

John W. Georgitis, MD

Director of Allergy, Immunology and Pediatric Pulmonary
Professor of Pediatrics
Bowman Gray School of Medicine
Winston-Salem, North Carolina

b

**Blackwell
Science**

Blackwell Science

Editorial offices:

Commerce Place, 350 Main Street, Malden,
  Massachusetts 02148, USA
Osney Mead, Oxford OX2 0El, England
25 John Street, London WC1N 2BL, England
23 Ainslie Place, Edinburgh EH3 6AJ, Scotland
54 University Street, Carlton, Victoria 3053,
  Australia
Other Editorial offices:
Arnette Blackwell SA, 224, Boulevard Saint
  Germain, 75007 Paris, France
Blackwell Wissenschafts-Verlag GmbH
  Kurfürstendamm 57, 10707 Berlin, Germany
Zehetnergasse 6, A-1140 Vienna, Austria

Distributors:

USA
Blackwell Science, Inc.
Commerce Place
350 Main Street
Malden, Massachusetts 02148
(Telephone orders: 800-215-1000 or
              617-388-8250;
      fax orders: 617-388-8270)

Canada
Copp Clark, Ltd.
2775 Matheson Blvd. East
Mississauga, Ontario
Canada, L4W 4P7
(Telephone orders: 800-263-4374 or
              905-238-6074)

Australia
Blackwell Science Pty. Ltd.
54 University Street
Carlton, Victoria 3053
03-9347-0300;
(Telephone orders: 03-9347-0300;
      fax orders: 03-9349-3016)

Outside North America and Australia
Blackwell Science, Ltd.
c/o Marston Book Services, Ltd.
P.O. Box 269
Abingdon
Oxon OX14 4YN
England
(Telephone orders: 44-01235-465500;
      fax orders: 44-01235-465555)

Acquisitions: Chris Davis
Development: Kathleen Broderick
Production: Irene Herlihy
Manufacturing: Lisa Flanagan
Typeset by Best-set Typesetter Ltd., Hong Kong
Printed and bound by BookCrafters
©1997 by Robert K. Bush and John
  W. Georgitis
Printed in the United States of America
96 97 98 99 5 4 3 2 1

Library of Congress Cataloging-in-Publication
Data
Bush, Robert K.
    Handbook of asthma and rhinitis/Robert K.
  Bush, John Georgitis.
        p.   cm.
    Includes bibliographical references and index.
    ISBN 0-86542-433-0 (alk. paper)
    1. Asthma.   2. Rhinitis.   I. Georgitis,
John.   II. Title.
    [DNLM: 1. Asthma—therapy. 2. Rhinitis.
WF 553 B978h 1997]
RC591.B87 1997
616.2'38—dc20
DNLM/DLC
for Library of Congress   96-42504
                                            CIP

*P*o 01059
15/7/97

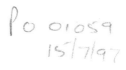
Coventry University

Contents

Preface

In 1995, Doctors William Busse and Stephen Holgate published an authoritative textbook, *Asthma and Rhinitis*, which is considered by many as the definitive work in the field. We, the authors of the *Handbook of Asthma and Rhinitis*, have abridged and modified many of the chapters from *Asthma and Rhinitis* to produce a clinically useful reference for the practitioner. Our purpose is to provide a succinct guide to the management of asthma and rhinitis. In addition, we have included relevant information regarding the pathophysiology and pharmacology of these conditions that formulate the basis of their treatment. In the constantly changing area of therapeutics, new approaches are discussed that may enter clinical practice in the near future. Attention is directed at specific problems encountered in clinical practice, including management of asthma in children, acute exacerbations in adults, exercise-induced asthma, nocturnal asthma, aspirin-sensitive asthma, and immunotherapy in the treatment of allergic disease. We feel that the *Handbook of Asthma and Rhinitis* will not only be of practical interest for the primary care physician, but will also be useful to the specialist in respiratory diseases.

We wish to thank the support of our families and the dedication of the staff of Blackwell Science who helped make this handbook possible.

R.K.B.
J.W.G.

Notice

The indications and dosages of all drugs in this book have been recommended in the medical literature and conform to the practices of the general medical community. The medications described do not necessarily have specific approval by the U.S. Food and Drug Administration for use in the diseases and dosages for which they are recommended. The package insert for each drug should be consulted for use and dosage as approved by the FDA. Because standards for usage change, it is advisable to keep abreast of revised recommendations, particularly those concerning new drugs.

Asthma

Introduction

CLINICAL DESCRIPTIONS AND DEFINITIONS

Asthma affects about 10% of the population, and its prevalence appears to be rising. There is concern that deaths from asthma are also increasing, but the reasons for this are unclear. There is even suspicion that some asthma therapies may be contributing to the increase in deaths. Some readers might be excused for thinking that asthma is a clearly defined disorder about which we can obtain information with confidence, but this is far from reality.

Evolution of the definition of asthma

Initially, asthma was the name given to the disorder occurring in people with "difficult breathing," especially of an episodic kind. This diagnosis did nothing to advance understanding, but it helped communication: one word conjured up this clinical presentation. When it was later shown that in some patients, left ventricular failure could account for this presentation, asthma was subdivided into two types—cardiac and bronchial. In time, as the nature of the circulatory changes secondary to left ventricular failure became clearer, better terms became available and the term *cardiac asthma* was dropped; bronchial asthma tended to become known simply as asthma.

Astute clinicians continued to make further observations on patients with asthma, observations which identified and increased understanding of its features. For example, nocturnal dyspnea has only relatively recently been recognized as a common feature of asthma; exercise-induced asthma was not clearly documented until 1966, yet today it has become an important diagnostic feature, especially in the young. Even cough has been recognized as the main presenting feature of asthma in some patients.

The introduction of simple methods of quantifying airflow obstruction focused attention on its reversibility, spontaneously or in response to therapy, in patients with attacks of asthma. They also permitted measurement of the response of the bronchi to inhaled agents such as histamine and demonstrated the high prevalence of increased reactivity of the bronchi in asthma. Similarly, demonstration of allergic and immunological changes in many but not all patients increased our knowledge and our uncertainties about asthma.

We have learned so much about the features of patients diagnosed with asthma that it may be surprising that we are unable to select features which all asthmatics have in common and therefore to agree on their use as operational criteria for the diagnosis. The explanation is simple: we have not yet identified features common to all patients we diagnose as having asthma.

Consider some of the features commonly encountered in asthma. This list is not meant to be exhaustive, only illustrative.

Reversible airflow obstruction: Otherwise normal patients who experience episodic attacks of breathlessness associated with wheezing are likely to be labeled or diagnosed as having "asthma." When these attacks are accompanied by objective measurement of markedly reversible airflow obstruction, they are the cardinal feature supporting the diagnosis. A definition based largely on this feature has been proposed: "Asthma is a disease characterized by wide variation over short periods of time in resistance to flow in the airways of the lung" (Ciba Foundation, Conference in London, 1959).

A major deficiency of this definition is that it is not written in operational terms that could allow one to decide unequivocally whether the defining features are present or not. For example, it does not state the degree of reversibility necessary, nor how the reversibility should be measured and expressed (i.e., what constitutes reversibility?).

But, just as unsatisfactorily, the term *asthma* is often applied to some patients with chronic, poorly reversible airflow obstruction.

Chronic airflow obstruction but with response to "anti-asthmatic" therapy: Unfortunately, patients presenting with reversible airflow obstruction sometimes progress to chronic irreversible airflow obstruction. This outcome seems to be more likely in patients with late-onset intrinsic asthma who are still liable to exacerbations with episodic worsening of their symptoms and continue to require the same treatment with antiasthmatic drugs such as sodium cromoglycate and/or corticosteroids. Although these patients no longer show marked reversibility, we still label their condition "asthma," but our reasons for doing so are different. Now we do so because they appear to have underlying disease processes that are similar, as judged by their response to treatment, but which present in different ways because the airways are no longer capable of the same degree of reversibility. Clinical features of irreversible airflow obstruction are superimposed and change the clinical presentation.

Clearly, reversibility *per se* is currently not a *sine qua non* for the diagnosis of asthma as currently applied. It is worth adding that patients with chronic airflow obstruction associated with chronic bronchitis and emphysema may show reversibility of the same order of magnitude, yet we are careful to differentiate these conditions from asthma largely because they do not respond clinically to these antiasthma drugs.

Pathological features: Are there any pathological features common to all asthmatics? For example, patients very commonly have eosinophils in the sputum and bronchi; these patients are also most likely to respond to therapy with anti-inflammatory drugs, which suggests common underlying mechanisms. However, there are patients, including those with certain types of occupational asthma, who do not fit this pattern.

When we consider other features that have been described in asthmatics, we find that no single feature or group of features is common to them all. So at present there are no exclusive defining characteristics that apply to all patients about whom we currently make this diagnosis. The majority of patients either possess a considerable degree of reversibility of airflow obstruction or are clearly responsive to anti-inflammatory agents; the majority have eosinophilia of the bronchial wall and its secretions, but apart from these the many other features tend to occur less regularly. We could make the arbitrary decision to define asthma by using these three features, but would it be an advantage? Some subjects currently included would be omitted, yet they might contain clues to better understanding of the nature of asthma.

The alternative is not to be restrictive but to describe in as much detail as possible the features of each of the patients being reported whenever they may need to be compared with other patients given the same diagnosis. This is essential if others are to be able to assess the significance of their results.

Perhaps one day we will decide that the word *asthma* no longer provides any advantage, and we may discard it—as we have done with *cardiac asthma*—or we may agree to restrict it only to patients with certain features.

Whatever we decide, or whatever new information we acquire to help us, the nature of the definition of asthma will not change—the meaning of the word *asthma* will always be what we choose it to be. We can only hope that this will reflect a far better understanding than we have at present of the processes that underlie the range of clinical presentations encompassed by "asthma."

For the clinician such developments would permit a more confident diagnostic and management approach; they would facilitate the application of agreed protocols of treatment and discourage inappropriate therapy with potentially harmful drugs. For the epidemiologist and those who conduct clinical trials, it would provide identification of a more homogeneous group of patients for study. For the more basic clinical scientist—physiologist, pharmacologist, pathologist, immunologist, or geneticist—it would provide a more homogeneous group for study with the likelihood of fewer confounding variables. But until we reach this happy state, if we ever do, we have no alternative but to strive to gain a greater understanding of the processes that interact with our bronchi to cause asthma.

MECHANISMS AND CLINICAL ASPECTS: AN OVERVIEW

This section is concerned with clinical aspects of asthma, focusing on three rather different problems: exercise-induced asthma, viral infections, and management. All are important in different ways.

Exercise-induced asthma

Exercise-induced asthma is important because of its social consequences, particularly for children, and because of the light it sheds on the pathophysiology of asthma. At least 80% of children with asthma bronchoconstrict following a standardized free-running exercise test, and many children and adults develop bronchoconstriction during and after exercise. In most instances the bronchoconstriction can be largely prevented by prior treatment with a β-agonist, sodium cromoglycate, or nedocromil, but there is evidence that exercise-induced asthma is often not managed particularly well. There is also evidence that asthmatic patients are less fit than they could be. These deficiencies in management can be attributed to failure to elicit information about problems with sporting activities and insufficient emphasis on preventative aspects of treatment. Restrictive attitudes and practices about the use of inhalers is a problem in some schools. One survey showed that teachers feel poorly prepared to supervise the management of children with asthma, are unduly worried about problems with inhalers, and are often uncertain as to whether children with asthma should be encouraged to participate in sports or not. More education of teachers and parents about asthma and sports is needed. The fact that several Olympic medal winners have had asthma should encourage children with asthma who wish to take part in competitive sports to do so.

Attempting to understand the pathophysiological changes in the airways that cause exercise-induced asthma has been pursued vigorously in recent years following the important observation that the magnitude of exercise-induced bronchoconstriction is related to heat loss across the airways. A series of elegant experiments in asthmatic patients involving inhalation of air of varying temperature and humidity during and after exercise and isocapnic hypopnea has shown that the magnitude of bronchoconstriction is related to water loss from the respiratory tract. How the water loss causes bronchoconstriction is the subject of some controversy. One theory argues a pivotal role for the bronchial circulation, water loss from the airways causing airway cooling and vasoconstriction of the bronchial vessels. When exercise stops, rapid rewarming of the airways causes vascular hyperemia and engorgement and airway narrowing. An opposing view argues that the crucial change is the increased osmolarity of the periciliary fluid caused by the evaporative water loss. The increased osmolarity causes mediator release from mast cells and possibly other cells, and these in turn cause airway smooth-muscle contraction, edema, and increased blood flow. The first hypothesis requires that airway cooling and rewarming occur whereas the second argues that these are not prerequisites for exercise-induced bronchoconstriction (Figure 1-1).

The main experimental findings and observations that favor airway cooling and rewarming as the cause of vascular hyperemia and airways obstruction are 1) the fact that breathing colder air after exercise reduces bronchoconstriction whereas breathing hot

Exercise-Induced Asthma

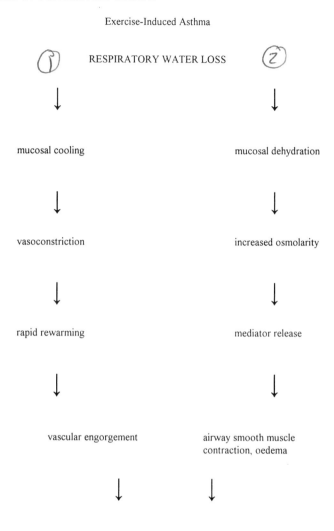

RESPIRATORY WATER LOSS

mucosal cooling · mucosal dehydration

vasoconstriction · increased osmolarity

rapid rewarming · mediator release

vascular engorgement · airway smooth muscle contraction, oedema

AIRWAY NARROWING

Figure 1-1. Outline of the two main hypotheses to explain exercise-induced asthma. (See text.)

air increases it, and 2) the fact that when airway temperature was measured, asthmatic airways rewarmed more rapidly than non-asthmatic airways. In addition, various maneuvers designed to increase or decrease bronchial blood flow (saline infusion, antishock trousers, noradrenaline treatment) were shown to attenuate or accentuate exercise-induced asthma. The hypothesis that increased osmolarity causes mediator release and airway narrowing is supported by the observation that in severe exercise-induced asthma bronchoconstriction may occur during rather than after exercise, by experiments which suggest that dry-air breathing causes vasodilation, not vasoconstriction, and by the fact that hot dry air causes bronchoconstriction even when expired temperature is high (airway temperature further down the airways is assumed to be relatively high). The ability of drugs such as sodium cromoglycate to inhibit exercise-induced asthma appears to favor the osmotic hypothesis as does a study using gases with different volume/heat capacities but similar water-carrying capacities (SF_6O_2 and HeO_2) which showed that bronchoconstriction is related to evaporative heat loss rather than total heat loss. Much of the evidence for both hypotheses is indirect in the sense that the mechanism of action of drugs such as sodium cromoglycate has not been established and treatments such as saline infusion are likely to have many effects other than a direct effect on the bronchial circulation. Direct measurement of airway temperature is obviously difficult and relatively crude. At present the precise mechanism of exercise-induced asthma remains unknown.

Viral infection

Viral infections are clearly important in asthma although how important is still uncertain. They are potentially relevant in three ways. First, they cause acute exacerbations of asthma and are the commonest cause of such attacks in young children. Second, some viruses, such as respiratory syncytial virus, cause a wheezing illness in young children which mimics asthma but does not necessarily develop into asthma. Third, and potentially the most important, is the possibility that a viral infection might in some way initiate asthma in those who are genetically predisposed.

Studies that have tried to identify and culture viruses during an exacerbation of asthma have provided a very variable yield, usually under 20% in adults with a rather higher figure, up to 50%, in young children. The extent to which the low figure in some series is due to problems in isolating viruses from the respiratory tract is uncertain. Use of the polymerase chain reaction to identify viral mRNA should help to determine more accurately the proportion of exacerbations that are due to a viral infection.

Recent studies have started to look at how viral infections

9

may cause exacerbations of asthma. Some viral infections such as respiratory syncytial virus, parainfluenza virus, and rhinovirus are associated with an increase in virus-specific IgE and with release of mast cell– or basophil-derived mediators such as tryptase. Experimental rhinovirus infection increases airway responsiveness to histamine and the early and late response to antigen challenge. Segmental antigen challenge carried out through a bronchoscope shows a pattern of release of cells, mediator, and cytokines in lavage fluid that suggests enhanced mast cell degranulation during the early response with subsequent accumulation of eosinophils and cytokines. Virus infection can affect the function of epithelial cells, inflammatory cells, and neural reflexes in a variety of ways.

If viral infections are an important cause of exacerbations in asthma, is immunization against viral infections safe, and would it be effective? Killed and attenuated influenza vaccine has been well tolerated in asthmatic patients, but how efficacious it is in reducing asthma morbidity is uncertain. Immunization against rhinovirus, the virus most commonly associated with exacerbations of asthma, is not available as yet.

Viral infections in children are common, and most recover without any long-term airway effects. Why then do some children develop persistent wheezing and increased bronchial responsiveness? Does the viral infection cause long-term effects on the airways, or is the viral infection seen as being more troublesome in children genetically predisposed to wheezing and bronchial hyperresponsiveness? The answers to these questions are not known and await detailed prospective studies of a cohort of children studied before and after viral infections. One hypothesis has been advanced that an immature or "dysregulated" immune system in young children could be responsible for an exaggerated response to some viral infections by causing increased production of IgE, a decrease in protective IgA and IgG, and overproduction or overactivity of cytotoxic T-cells, but this remains to be proven.

Management

At present asthma and allergic rhinitis cannot be cured, nor are there clear strategies for prevention. A reduction in maternal smoking should reduce the incidence of asthma, and allergen avoidance strategies in prenatal or early life may help, but these ideas need to be confirmed. Avoidance measures will reduce episodes of asthma for some patients, but the ubiquitous house dust mite is difficult to avoid. Most patients require some form of pharmacotherapy intermittently or on a regular basis.

Use of drugs: There are in essence only five groups of drugs that are widely used in asthma, and these can be divided broadly into bronchodilators (β-agonists, theophyllines, and to a lesser extent, antimuscarinic drugs) and prophylactic drugs (corticosteroids, sodium cromoglycate, and nedocromil). This division is slightly artificial as β-agonists, for example, prevent exercise-induced asthma and corticosteroids cause bronchodilation, though over days rather than hours. The aim of treatment is to provide symptomatic relief and freedom from acute attacks of asthma without causing side effects or long-term health problems such as osteoporosis. The art of managing asthma lies in being able to juggle the treatment to provide the best balance of benefit compared to side effects and long-term risk in an individual patient.

There are large international differences in the sale and use of various drugs for asthma, much of which are unexplained. Inhaled steroids, for example, account for 45% (by cost) of sales in the United Kingdom, 14% in the United States, and 5% in Japan. There is no evidence to suggest that asthmatic patients in various countries respond differently to these drugs, and this is inherently unlikely. The implication, therefore, is that our methods of determining the effectiveness of treatment are still poor and that doctors prescribing drugs are being overly influenced by market forces rather than pharmacological considerations. The same is almost certainly true for rhinitis, though there are fewer data.

Assessing side effects: Determining the acute effects and side effects of drugs is usually not very difficult, particularly for rapidly acting drugs such as bronchodilators. Two areas cause particular difficulty in the assessment of antiasthma treatment. First is the assessment of long-term side effects such as the possible increase in osteoporosis that might occur with inhaled steroids twenty or thirty years after treatment is started. At present, proxy measures of the likely development of osteoporosis such as bone mineral density are being used, but it will be difficult to quantify the risk accurately, and physicians' perception of the risk is likely to vary considerably. The second difficulty is assessing the risk of consequences that may be severe or even fatal but occur very rarely. Assuming the relation to be causal, the number of deaths in relation to the number of patients taking β-agonists is extremely small, and such a relationship could be picked up only by a very large prospective study. It has been estimated, for example, that 75,000 patients would need to be studied for four months with a new β-agonist to detect a twofold increase in mortality compared to albuterol.

Management (as opposed to treatment): A major development over the last ten years has been the introduction of guidelines for the management of asthma and a shift towards patients adjusting their treatment more, within certain boundaries. The guidelines emphasize a stepwise approach, with treatment increasing from an occasional β-agonist for patients with intermittent symptoms at one end to the addition of oral corticosteroids to inhaled corticosteroids, β-agonists, and antimuscarinic drugs in patients with severe disease at the other. The role of inhaled steroids at an early stage of the disease is emphasized strongly. The guidelines have a useful role in emphasizing the importance of altering treatment as symptoms dictate, particularly for physicians less familiar with asthma. There are legitimate concerns, however, that they may provide an intellectual straitjacket or be adhered to rigidly in situations where they are inappropriate. They are essentially guidelines for nonexperts, and represent a consensus view at the time they were written. Most of the recommendations are based on experience and have not been formally tested.

The introduction of personal action plans for patients recognizes the need for flexible and rapid adjustment of treatment for such a variable disease as asthma. Patients are encouraged to adjust their medication within specified boundaries according to their symptoms and, in many countries, peak flow rate. The plan should include clear instructions about what the patient should do as and when his or her asthma deteriorates. Asthma nurses are playing a more prominent role in many countries, being more available than doctors and well able to advise patients about increasing and decreasing treatment, again within predetermined limits. The guidelines also suggest when specialist help should be sought: for patients who have severe acute attacks or whose symptoms are not controlled by inhaled drugs, for example, and those with aspirin-sensitive or occupational asthma.

New drugs: With the exception of leukotriene receptor antagonists, the long-acting β-agonists salmeterol and formoterol are the only new drugs introduced for asthma in the last five years. They are clearly effective, though the extent to which this is due to their long duration of action, the dose administered, or other actions is still uncertain. More information is required on their pharmacological profile and long-term effects.

Several new classes of drugs are currently under investigation in humans. There is considerable interest in mediator antagonists, including antagonists of platelet activating factor (PAF), thromboxane, and leukotriene and 5-lipoxygenase inhibitors. The results with PAF and thromboxane antagonists have been disappointing, but the new generation of leukotriene antagonists looks considerably more promising than the early drugs and are now available for clinical use. Several have now caused some bronchodilatation in acute studies and marked inhibition of exercise and antigen challenge. The results of longer-term treatment of asthma are awaited. So far, the potassium channel activators have been disappointing, and drugs with a more selective action on airway cells are required if beneficial effects are to be dissociated from side effects. The same is true for calcium antagonists.

Steroid-sparing drugs such as methotrexate, gold salts, and, more recently, cyclosporin allow patients with severe asthma to reduce the dose of oral corticosteroid. All have side effects, however, and whether the number of side effects that would accrue over many years from these drugs is greater or less than the number saved by a relatively modest reduction in oral corticosteroid dose is uncertain.

Although theophylline is an effective bronchodilator in asthma, it has to be given orally and its value is limited by variable metabolism among subjects and a small therapeutic window. There is still some uncertainty about how theophylline works and the extent to which its bronchodilator activity is related to phosphodiesterase inhibition. Five different phosphodiesterase enzymes have been identified, and the development of more specific enzyme inhibitors holds the promise of drugs with a more selective action on the airways and fewer side effects. These drugs are currently under investigation in patients.

The role of the excitatory nonadrenergic noncholinergic nerve supply to human airways is uncertain. If it is important in asthma, neurokinin antagonists such as FK224 may have a therapeutic role; this possibility is now being investigated.

Inhalation of furosemide inhibits the bronchoconstrictor response to stimuli that act indirectly on the airways such as exercise, allergens, and sodium metabisulfite. Understanding the mechanism whereby furosemide causes these effects is of interest in understanding the pathophysiology of asthma. Whether furosemide will have a therapeutic role is less certain since in many respects it resembles sodium cromoglycate, and it may not have any advantages over sodium cromoglycate.

A wide range of drugs with different modes of action is currently under investigation for the treatment of asthma and rhinitis, holding out the possibility of new therapeutic approaches in the future. In parallel with this are studies looking at drugs in current use, such as β-agonists and corticosteroids, to understand better their mode of action so that new drugs with greater efficacy and fewer side effects can be produced. There is at present enormous activity with considerable diversity in approach. Although there is a large jump between demonstrating therapeutic efficacy in animal models and producing an effective drug for patients, it is to be hoped that some at least of the many drugs currently under investigation will achieve that jump.

SELECTED REFERENCES

Beasley R, Burgess C, Crane J, Pearce N, Roche W. Pathology of asthma and its clinical implications. J Allergy Clin Immunol 1993;92:148–154.

Cypcar D, Busse WW. Role of viral infections in asthma. Immunol Allergy Clin No. Amer 1993;13:745–768.

Eggleston PA. Exercise-induced asthma. In: Bierman CW, Pearlman DS, Shapiro GC, Busse WW, eds. Allergy, asthma, and immunology from infancy to adulthood. 3rd ed. Philadelphia: W.B. Saunders, 1996:520–528.

Seaton A, Godden DJ, Brown K. Increase in asthma: a more toxic environment or a more susceptible population? Thorax 1994;49:171–174.

Toelle BG, Peat JK, Salome CM, Mellis CM, Woolcock AJ. Towards a definition of asthma for epidemiology. Am Rev Respir Dis 1992;146:633–637.

The Role of House Dust Mites and Other Allergens in Asthma

2

INTRODUCTION

Numerous antigens—including but not limited to dust mites, pollens, and fungi and those derived from insects or other animals—are capable of triggering acute attacks of asthma. Further studies clearly show a very strong correlation between exposure and sensitization to indoor allergens and the development of asthma. As a result, allergen avoidance should now be considered an integral part of the management of asthma. Rigid allergen avoidance might also prevent the development of asthma in genetically susceptible individuals, but there are no published studies to support this notion directly.

The causal role of house dust mites in asthma is emphasized because it is the most critically studied. However, numerous other allergens (Table 2-1) can be important triggers of acute attacks and may also be important in initiating or maintaining the underlying inflammation and bronchial hyperresponsiveness (BHR), which characterize asthma (Figure 2-1).

HOUSE DUST MITES

Mites are arthropods of the order Acari. The term "house dust mites" designates species of the family Pyroglyphidae that occur frequently in house dust, four of which are dominant: *Dermatophagoides pteronyssinus*, *D. farinae*, *D. microceras*, and *Euroglyphus*

Table 2-1. Structural and Functional Properties of Indoor Allergens

Source	Allergen[a]	Molecular weight (kDa)	Function	Sequence[b]
House dust mite				
Dermatophagoides spp.	Group 1	25	Cysteine protease	cDNA
	Group 2	14	Unknown	cDNA
	Group 3	~30	Serine protease	Protein
	Der p 4	~60	Amylase	Protein
	Der p 5	14	Unknown	cDNA
	Der p 6	25	Chymotrypsin	Protein
	Der p 7	22–28	Unknown	cDNA
Euroglyphus maynei	*Eur m 1*	25	Cysteine protease	PCR
Blomia tropicalis	*Blo t 5*	14	Unknown	cDNA
Lepidoglyphus destructor	*Lep d 1*	14	Unknown	None
Mammals				
Felis domesticus	*Fel d 1*	36	(Uteroglobin)	PCR
Canis familiaris	*Can f 1*	25	Unknown	cDNA
Mus musculus	*Mus m 1*	19	Calycine, pheromone	cDNA
Rattus norvegicus	*Rat n 1*	19	Binding proteins	cDNA
Cockroach				
Blattella germanica	*Bla g 1*	20–25	Unknown	None
	Bla g 2	36	Aspartic protease	cDNA
	Bla g 4	21	Calycine	cDNA
	Bla g 5	36	Glutathione transferase	cDNA
Periplaneta americana	*Per a 1*	20–25	Unknown	None
	Per a 3	72–78	Unknown	None
Fungi				
Aspergillus fumigatus	*Asp f 1*	18	Cytotoxin (mitogillin)	cDNA

[a] New nomenclature proposed by the WHO/IUIS subcommittee.
[b] Method given for full sequence determination, where available. However, protein sequences are incomplete; usually N-terminal or internal peptide sequences have been determined.
SOURCE: Chapman MD, Heymann PW, Sporik RB, Platts-Mills TAE. Monitoring allergic exposure in asthma: new treatment strategies. Allergy 1995;50(25):29–33 (with permission).

maynei. *D. pteronyssinus* and *E. maynei* are more common in Europe, while *D. farinae* is equally common in North America. Other species, usually regarded as storage mites, do occur in houses. *Blomia tropicalis*, found in house dust in tropical or semi-tropical areas, is not easily classified as either a storage mite or Pyroglyphid. These species are important because they are present in large numbers in domestic houses and because extracts made from cultures of these mites can elicit skin test responses and radioallergosorbent test (RAST) activity. Optimal growth of house dust mites requires high humidity, moderate temperature (70 to 80°F), and adequate food sources (human skin scales). The largest

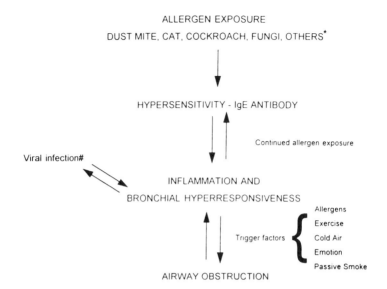

Figure 2-1. Etiology of asthma and airway hyperresponsiveness.
* Seasonal pollens, occupational allergens, ? others
\# Viral infection can either directly contribute to bronchial hyperresponsiveness or act to increase the response to allergen exposure

numbers of mites are usually found in dust samples taken from uncovered mattress surfaces, bedding, upholstered furniture, and floor carpeting. However, other locations such as stuffed toys, clothing, and drapes can also be important mite habitats. Seasonal variations in mite level occur mainly in carpets and other places where drying occurs relatively rapidly.

Considerable progress has been made in the purification, identification, and definition of individual mite allergens. Three groups of mite allergens have been defined and are designated Group I, II, and III allergens. The Group I allergens (*Der p 1*, *Der f 1*, and *Eur m 1*) are proteases of approximate molecular weight 25,000, which are secreted from the digestive tract and found in high concentration in mite feces. Group II allergens (*Der p 2*, *Der f 2*) are found in both fecal pellets and mite bodies. Their function is unknown. Over 80% of mite allergic patients have IgE antibodies to Group I and II allergens. Group III allergens (*Der p 3*, *Der f 3*) are also digestive enzymes; however, the quantity of Group III allergens in house dust is at least one log lower than that of Group I and II allergens. Only about 20% of mite allergic individuals have IgE antibodies to Group III allergens. Group I mite allergens have approximately 75% amino acid homology within the group; and, as judged by IgE antibodies, there is moderate cross-reactivity. By contrast, most monoclonal antibodies raised against *Der p 1* or *Der f 1* are species specific. Group II allergens demonstrate a greater degree of cross-reactivity with both IgE and monoclonal antibodies and have approximately 85% amino acid sequence homology within the group. There is no cross-reactivity or sequence homology between Group I and Group II allergens. Many other components of dust mite extracts bind IgE antibodies, one of which is a 60-kDa protein (mite amylase) purified from *D. pteronyssinus*. The importance of these other allergens remains to be determined.

Sensitization and exposure to house dust mites

House dust mite allergens seem to be particularly immunogenic. In areas of high exposure, it appears that virtually all potentially atopic children become sensitized to mite antigens by age fourteen. Although it can occur at any age, predisposed individuals appear more susceptible to sensitization during infancy. Evidence from a number of studies supports the idea that sensitization to allergens is dependent on the level of exposure in a dose-dependent fashion. This has led to the proposal of threshold levels of exposure above which sensitization becomes increasingly more likely. For house dust mites, this proposed level is $2\,\mu g$ of Group I allergen per gram of dust (Table 2-2). Exposure of sensitized individuals to levels greater than $10\,\mu g$ of Group I allergen per gram of dust increases the risk of acute asthma attacks. However, the evidence for a dose-response relationship to symptoms is less complete than for sensitization. Once sensitization to inhalant allergens develops, it usually persists into adult life.

House dust mites as a cause of asthma

There are several studies which show an association between sensitization to dust mite allergens and asthma. In a cohort of children in New Zealand, there was a highly significant association between dust mite sensitization and the development of asthma. Case control studies from around the world have confirmed the association in mite allergic subjects. A prospective study in the United King-

Table 2-2. Proposed Threshold Values for Indoor Allergens

| | Exposure leading to | |
	IgE sensitization	Allergic symptoms
Dust mite		
Group 1 allergen	$>2\,\mu g/g$	$10\,\mu g/g\star$
Mite counts	$>100\,mites/g$	>500 mites/g$\star$
Guanine	$>0.9\,mg/g$	$>3.0\,mg/g$
Cat—Fel d 1	$>8\,\mu g/g$	?
	1–$8\,\mu g/g$	?
Dog—Can f 1	$>10\,\mu g/g$	?
Cockroach—Bla g 2	$>2\,units/g$	?

$\star$ A level above which patients who are going to develop symptoms will do so. This level increases the risk of acute asthma.
SOURCE: Chapman MD, Heymann PW, Sporik RB, Platts-Mills TAE. Monitoring allergic exposure in asthma: new treatment strategies. Allergy 1995;50(25):29–33 (with permission).

dom demonstrated that exposure to greater than $10\,\mu g$ of mite allergen per gram of dust in early childhood was an important predictor of the development of asthma by age eleven. Additionally, studies of patients presenting to emergency rooms with acute asthma have demonstrated significant associations with dust mite sensitization and exposure.

A causal role for mite exposure in asthma is further supported by evidence that the prevalence of the disease is lower in areas of low mite exposure such as among native Inuit, children raised at high altitude in Europe, and highland natives of Papua New Guinea. Furthermore, decreased exposure to mite allergens has been shown to result in improvement of symptoms and decreased BHR. While inhalation of allergens cannot explain all cases of asthma, it does seem to be of primary importance in the development of the disease in many children and young adults. Thus, allergen avoidance should be a primary treatment for asthma in allergic patients.

Dust mite avoidance and immunotherapy

With recent advances in the measurement of mite allergen levels in houses, it is now possible to assess the efficacy of various avoidance regimes. Many measures have been shown to be effective in reducing mite levels (Table 2-3). Encasement of mattresses, box springs, and pillows in zippered plastic or vapor-permeable fabrics is very

Table 2-3. Control Measures—Dust Mites

- Encase mattress and pillows
- Wash bedclothes weekly at 130°F ($\geq$54°C)
- Reduce indoor relative humidity to $\leq$50%
- ? Apply tannic acid solution to carpets or upholstered furniture
- ? Apply acaracide

effective. Removal of carpeting, especially in the bedroom, has likewise been shown to be effective. Washing bedding in hot water (130°F) can kill mites and is usually recommended every ten to fourteen days. Reduction of indoor humidity may also be helpful in controlling mite growth. A variety of chemicals can reduce mite levels, including acaricides such as benzyl benzoate and protein-denaturing agents such as tannic acid, which inactivate the allergens. The role of these chemicals and the optimal methods of application need further clarification. Simple vacuum cleaning is not effective in removing live mites. The filtration efficiency of different models of vacuum cleaners varies widely, and some vacuum cleaners can actually increase airborne mite allergen levels. Central or room air cleaners are of little value. Trials of dust avoidance in sensitized asthmatic children have shown decreased bronchial responsiveness to histamine, symptom improvement, and decreased medication use in the treated group. Significant reduction of BHR has also been shown in adults admitted to an "allergen-free" environment in a hospital, although this required two to three months. In the long run it will be necessary to design and maintain houses so as to prevent mite infestation.

There are conflicting but generally favorable reports on the efficacy of immunotherapy for asthma related to house dust mites. Its use can be considered in patients who do not respond adequately to avoidance measures and simple medications. Deciding which asthmatics are the best candidates for immunotherapy is, however, difficult as the more severe patients are more likely to experience serious adverse reactions. Therefore, allergen immunotherapy should be undertaken carefully and should be administered only by physicians with the appropriate training and expertise.

COCKROACHES

Cockroach sensitization may be more important than that to dust mites among inner-city asthmatics in the northern United States. Both immediate and late responses to bronchial challenge have been documented. Additional studies from around the U.S. have confirmed a high prevalence of IgE antibody to cockroach allergens among asthmatic patients. Cockroaches have also been reported to cause asthma in other parts of the world and to cause occupational allergy among laboratory workers. Emergency room studies have revealed that sensitization and exposure to cockroaches is a major risk factor for acute asthma among African-American patients.

The most common species are *Blatella germanica* (German cockroach) and *Perplaneta americana* (American cockroach). At least two allergens have been identified and defined from *B. germanica*, designated as *Bla g 1* and *Bla g 2*. There are undoubtedly more to be defined. Antigenic cross reactivity between species is poorly understood at this point. Enzyme-linked immunoabsorbent assay (ELISA) techniques to measure levels of *Bla g 1* or *Bla g 2* have been developed. The highest indoor levels of cockroach allergen are usually found on kitchen floors and in cabinets.

There is convincing evidence that cockroach allergy is important in some asthmatics, especially among patients living in poor housing conditions. Patients presenting for evaluation of asthma who live in houses that could be cockroach infested should be evaluated for cockroach sensitivity by skin or RAST testing. Avoidance measures (Table 2-4) and/or immunotherapy can be considered as part of their management, in addition to pharmacologic therapy. However, avoidance measures are not well defined, and there is still a need for evidence that avoidance measures and/or immunotherapy are effective in controlling symptoms in these patients.

Table 2-4.   Control Measures—Cockroaches

- Remove food sources
- Reduce access to water
- Seal access and entry points
- Spray runways with 0.5–1% diazinon or chlorpyrifor
- Blow boric acid powder under stoves, refrigerator
- Place bait stations (hydramethylnon) at feeding sites

CATS

Immediate sensitivity to cats is well documented among allergic patients. At least 2% of the population may be allergic to cats. Additionally, sensitization to cats is common among asthmatic patients. The combination of sensitization and exposure to cats has been shown to be an important risk factor for acute asthma. In contrast to cockroach sensitivity, cat sensitization is more common among suburban patients.

The major cat allergen, *Fel d 1*, is a 36-kDa glycoprotein found in saliva and sebaceous glands. Other proteins, such as cat albumin, are considered minor allergens. ELISA assays have been developed for measurement of *Fel d 1*. High levels of cat allergen can be found all over the house, on clothing, furniture, and floors. Patients who are allergic to cats typically report a rapid onset of symptoms after exposure. This probably is due to the fact that *Fel d 1* is commonly associated with particles less than 2.5 µm in diameter, which can remain airborne in undisturbed conditions. Low air-exchange rates, increased furnishings, and the cat itself play significant roles in increasing airborne cat allergen levels. When a cat was kept in a room with carpeting and upholstered furniture, the accumulation of *Fel d 1* was about 100 times greater than in the same room with polished floors and wooden furniture. The most obvious technique to reduce airborne allergen levels is removing the cat, either completely or outdoors (Table 2-5). The level of *Fel d 1* in dust falls slowly after removal of the cat and may persist for up to six months. Also passive transfer of cat allergen into a house on the clothing of occupants or visitors can produce significant levels in dust. If the cat cannot be removed, washing it weekly may be of benefit, although this is debatable. Allergen accumulates on the fur, mainly by coming directly through the skin. Distribution of allergen from salivary sources by the cat licking itself is probably less important than previously thought. Other measures to reduce

---

Table 2-5.   Control Measures—Cat in Situ

- Remove animal from bedroom
- Remove carpets
- Use HEPA (high-efficiency particulate air cleaner) filtered vacuum cleaner on floors
- Use high-efficiency room air cleaner
- ? Wash animal weekly
- ? Apply tannic acid solution to carpets

---

airborne levels of cat allergen include having polished floors instead of carpet, air filtration, vacuuming with a high-efficiency filter, and minimization of upholstered furnishings. Immunotherapy has limited effectiveness in the treatment of asthma related to cat allergy.

OTHER INDOOR ALLERGENS

There are many other allergens besides those from dust mites, cats, and cockroaches in houses that can contribute to asthma symptoms in a particular patient or area. Feathers have long been accepted as an important indoor allergen; however, it is unclear if feather allergy is due to actual bird-derived proteins or rather to the fact that mites, fungi, or other organisms can grow readily on feathers. Additional sources of allergens that can sometimes be found in houses include rodents (where urine is the major source of allergen), dogs or other mammals, various insects, and indoor fungi.

POLLEN

A variety of airborne pollens can act as allergens in atopic patients and cause clinical disease. Seasonal allergic rhinitis is obviously a major cause of morbidity in allergic patients, but asthma may also be exacerbated by exposure to pollens. Although pollen grains are typically described as being too large to reach the lung, a small fraction of large particles (approximately 5%) traverse the oropharynx and enter the airways, resulting in a local inflammatory response in the lung which contributes both to short-term obstruction and to longer-term bronchial irritability. Many grasses, trees, and weeds, particularly ragweed, have been implicated as triggers of acute asthma attacks. There are relatively few areas of the world where the number of cases of pollen-associated asthma is sufficient to allow conclusions to be drawn about the level of pollen exposure that is a risk factor for asthma. Because pollen can enter houses and the allergens may accumulate to high levels in house dust, a simple correlation with outdoor pollen counts cannot be expected. In certain areas a defined pollen season can be associated with an annual epidemic of asthma (e.g., grass pollen in California).

Methods of avoiding exposure to pollen have not been studied very well, but obvious techniques include minimizing time outdoors during the relevant season and use of air conditioning.

Immunotherapy has been shown to be an effective treatment for seasonal asthma related to ragweed and grass pollen and may be of benefit for other pollens as well.

FUNGI

Exposure to airborne spores and other fungal particles can induce immediate hypersensitivity and serum IgE antibodies in atopic subjects. Additionally, there is increasing evidence that fungi can be important causes of asthma.

In general, it has been difficult to establish the allergenic importance of airborne fungi. Investigation has been complicated by the fact that there are literally thousands of fungal species, many of which are reported to cause hypersensitivity reactions. Lack of strict seasonal patterns of exposure has also contributed to this difficulty. Furthermore, the highly variable expression of fungal allergens between strains from the same species or under different culture conditions has made it difficult to characterize specific allergens, and to date, very few fungal allergens have been purified.

In spite of this difficulty, at least five classes of fungi appear to have been implicated as sources of aeroallergens. These are Ascomycetes, Basidiomycetes, Deuteromycetes (Fungi Imperfecti), Oomycetes, and Zygomycetes. High levels of basidiospores have been correlated with asthma epidemics in the United States (New Orleans) and New Zealand. Subsequent studies have shown significant skin test reactivity to Basidiomycetes species in asthmatic patients in various parts of the world.

Numerous investigators have shown temporal relationships between respiratory symptoms and exposure to fungal allergens. One study demonstrated a correlation between outdoor fungal spore levels and low peak flow values and another has shown a correlation between *Cladosporium* levels and both symptoms and medication use in asthmatics with positive bronchial provocations and skin tests. Several epidemiological studies from the United States and Australia have implicated *Alternaria* sensitivity as a risk factor for asthma. Another investigation identified *Alternaria* exposure as a risk factor for respiratory arrest in young asthmatics. Thus it seems clear that, in sensitive patients, exposure to some airborne fungi and fungal elements may be an important trigger of asthma. Much remains to be learned about the tremendous number of species of fungi which can cause human disease and the nature of their allergens, as well as the efficacy of possible treatment regimes such as avoidance measures (Table 2-6) and immunotherapy.

In addition to airborne fungi, a fungal organism residing on the skin (the dermatophyte *Trichophyton*) can be an important source of sensitization and antigen exposure in some asthmatics. Specific antifungal therapy (funconazole) appears to be both safe and beneficial in these patients. Whether or not other fungi could act in a similar fashion remains to be assessed.

OCCUPATIONAL ASTHMA

Asthma related to the workplace has been reported with inhalational exposure to literally hundreds of substances, and the list continues to grow. Some examples are found in Tables 2-7 and 2-8. The agents implicated can induce asthma symptoms by either immunologic or nonimmunologic mechanisms. Classical IgE mediated immediate hypersensitivity has been described for many high molecular weight protein allergens derived from a variety of plants, insects or other animals, or bacteria. There are also low molecular weight chemicals that are capable of inducing IgE responses in some patients after combining with larger endogenous carrier proteins such as albumin. This mechanism appears to at least contribute to asthma occurring in workers with inhalational exposure to substances such as antibiotics, platinum salts, anhydrides, some diisocyanates, and possibly plicatic acid in Western red cedar dust. Other chemicals appear to act through nonimmunologic mechanisms such as reflex bronchoconstriction, irritation of bronchial epithelium, or direct pharmacologically induced bronchoconstriction. For example, cholinesterase-inhibiting organophosphate insecticides can cause bronchospasm in exposed

---

Table 2-6. Control Measures—Fungi

- Outdoor fungi
    - Close windows, use air conditioning
    - Avoid exposure to decaying vegetation (e.g., leaf raking)
    - Consider face mask
- Indoor fungi
    - Maintain indoor relative humidity at $\leq 50\%$
    - Clean washable surfaces with 5% bleach solution
    - Remove sources (e.g., contaminated carpets)

Table 2-7. Causes of Occupational Asthma: Allergic Mechanism, High Molecular Weight Compounds*

Agents	Examples	Industries
Lab animals	Rat, mouse, rabbit, guinea pig	Lab workers, veterinarians, animal handlers
Birds	Pigeon, chicken, budgerigar	Pigeon breeders, poultry workers, bird fanciers
Insects	Grain mite, locust	Grain workers, research lab staff
	River fly	Power plants along rivers
	Screwworm fly, cockroach, cricket	Flight crews, lab workers, field contacts
	Bee moth, moth, butterfly	Fish bait breeders, entomologists
Plants	Rubber plant (latex)	Health care workers, manufacturing
	Grain dust, wheat/rye flour	Grain handlers, bakers, millers
	Buckwheat, coffee bean, tobacco leaf	Bakers, food processors, tobacco manufacturing
	Castor bean, tea	Oil industry, teaworker
	Hops (*Humulus lupulus*)	Brewery chemists
Biologic enzymes	*B. subtilis*, trypsin, pancreatin	Detergent industry, plastic/ pharmaceutical, pharmaceutical
	Papain, pepsin, flaviastase, bromelin	Lab packaging, pharmaceutical
	Fungal amylase	Manufacturing, bakers
Vegetables	Gum acacia, gum tragacanth	Printers, gum manufacturing
Other	Crab, prawn, hoya, silkworm larva	Crab and prawn processing, oyster farm, sericulture

*Adapted with permission from Chan-Yeung M, Lam S. Am Rev Respir Dis 1986; 133:686–703.

workers. Numerous other inorganic and organic chemicals including diisocyanates, wood dusts, and others act through as yet uncertain mechanisms, and in some instances more than one mechanism may be involved. Toluene diisocyanate (TDI) has been shown in vitro to inhibit isoproterenol-induced cyclic AMP production by peripheral blood lymphocytes in a dose-related manner. TDI also acts as an irritant at high concentration. However, asthma occurs in only a small proportion (5 to 10%) of those exposed. In addition,

Table 2-8. Causes of Occupational Asthma: Allergic or Possibly Allergic Mechanism, Low Molecular Weight Compounds*

Agents	Examples	Industries
Diisocyanates	Toluene	Polyurethane industry, plastics, varnish
	Diphenylmethane, hexamethylene	Foundries, automobile spray painting
Anhydrides	Phthalic, trimellitic, tetrachlorophthalic	Epoxy resins, plastics
Wood dusts	Western red cedar, California redwood cedar of Lebanon, Cocabolla, Iroko oak, Mahogany, Abiruana, Kejaat African maple, Tanganyika aningre Central American walnut, African zebra wood	Carpentry, construction, cabinetmaking, sawmill
Metals	Platinum, nickel, chromium	Platinum refinery, metal plating, tanning
	Cobalt, vanadium, tungsten carbide	Hard metal industry
Fluxes	Aminoethyl ethanolamine, colophony	Aluminum soldering, electronics
Drugs	Penicillins, cephalosporins, psyllium	Pharmaceuticals, laxative manufacturer
	Phenylglycine acid chloride, spiramycin	Pharmaceuticals
	Piperazine hydrochloride, methyldopa	Chemist, pharmaceuticals
	Salbutamol intermediate, tetracycline	Pharmaceuticals
Other chemicals	Azodicarbonamide, formalin, freon	Plastics and rubber, hospital staff, refrigeration
	Dimethyl ethanolamine	Spray painting
	Persulfate salts and henna	Hairdressing
	Ethylene diamine	Photography
	Diazonium salt	Photocopying and dye
	Hexachlorophene (sterilizing agent)	Hospital staff
	Urea formaldehyde	Insulation, resin
	Paraphenylene diamine	Fur dying
	Furfural alcohol (furan-based resin)	Foundry mold making

*Adapted with permission from Chan-Yeung M, Lam S. Am Rev Respir Dis 1986; 133:686–703.

asthmatic symptoms can take weeks or months to develop after the onset of exposure and can be provoked by very low concentrations of TDI in sensitized subjects, suggesting a possible IgE-mediated immune mechanism.

In all instances of occupational asthma, the only rational treatment is complete avoidance of the offending agent. In many cases this necessitates a change of occupation. If the diagnosis is made and complete avoidance is instituted early enough, progression to severe refractory asthma can often be prevented. Pharmacologic treatment is necessary for acute episodes and is similar to treatment of nonoccupational asthma, but should not be used as a substitute for avoidance measures. On a broader scale, methods to reduce exposure of workers to potentially sensitizing agents (e.g., shielding, masks, and ventilation) need to be studied and implemented to prevent the development of the disease where possible.

CONCLUSION

It is now widely accepted that inflammation of the airways is a key component of asthma. It follows that there should be a primary stimulus driving this inflammation. Allergens certainly are capable of fulfilling this role. Epidemiologic data support a very strong correlation between immediate hypersensitivity to inhaled allergens and the development of asthma. The evidence is most complete regarding house dust mite allergens, but an increasing number of studies suggest that allergens derived from cats, cockroaches, and *Alternaria* are important as well.

The central roles of allergen sensitization/exposure and inflammation in the pathogenesis of asthma provide a rational basis for the use of anti-inflammatory drugs, immunotherapy, and immune-modifying drugs in selected patients. The primary therapeutic implication of the information presented herein, however, is that allergen avoidance is the logical first-line treatment for asthma in allergic patients. Avoidance is helpful in the management of symptomatic disease and may also be effective in preventing the onset of asthma in some susceptible infants.

SELECTED REFERENCES

Bernstein DI. Occupational asthma. Med Clin North Am 1992; 76:917–934.

DeBlay F, Chapman MD, Platts-Mills TAE. Airborne cat allergen (*Fel d 1*): environmental control with the cat *in situ*. Am Rev Respir Dis 1991;143:1334–1339.

Ingram JM, Heymann PW. Environmental controls in the management of asthma. Immunol Allergy Clin No Amer 1993;13:785.

O'Hollaren MT, Yunginger J, Offord KP, et al. Exposure to an aeroallergen as a possible precipitating factor in respiratory arrest in young patients with asthma. N Engl J Med 1991;324:359–363.

Platts-Mills TAE, Thomas WR, Aalberse RC, Vervloet D, Chapman MD. Dust mite allergens and asthma: report of a 2nd international workshop. J Allergy Clin Immunol 1992;89: 1046–1060.

Sporik R, Holgate ST, Platts-Mills TAE, Cogswell J. Exposure to house dust mite allergen (*Der p 1*) and the development of asthma in childhood: a prospective study. N Engl J Med 1990;323:502–507.

Treatment of Asthma

3

AIMS OF ASTHMA TREATMENT

Currently, the aims of the treatment of asthma are to prevent symptoms and to protect the patient from the long-term risks of the disease. The importance of preventing attacks has been stressed for a number of years, but it is only since the role of inflammation became widely appreciated that more precise aims have been introduced. Although it seems reasonable to aim to reduce the long-term risks of altered lifestyle, permanently altered lung function, the side effects of drugs, and premature death by controlling the airway inflammation as completely as possible, it is not known if currently available management allows these aims to be achieved.

A future aim of asthma treatment is to prevent the disease in the next generation of children. Since there is increasing evidence that persistent asthma is an incurable disease, prevention of the disease (not just its symptoms) is now becoming a matter of importance.

DEFINITIONS

Asthma

Asthma is a disease of the airways, characterized by chronic inflammation that makes them prone to narrow too easily and too much. Asthma is classified into several forms—episodic or seasonal (characterized by episodes of symptoms with essentially normal airway function between episodes), persistent (abnormal airway function in response to a wide range of provoking stimuli is present at all times), and obstructed (evidence of permanent airflow limitation between episodes of symptoms).

Acute exacerbations

An acute exacerbation of asthma is an episode of symptoms of varying duration and severity that requires treatment. This may vary from a mild wheeze, relieved by a bronchodilator, to status asthmaticus requiring treatment in hospital.

Airway hyperresponsiveness

Airway hyperresponsiveness (AHR) is a cardinal feature of asthma and is defined as an abnormal response to inhaled histamine or methacholine. A curve that lies outside the normal range (curves A to E in Figure 3-1) indicates an abnormality of the airway wall, but for the purposes of treatment, if the dose (concentration) that causes a 20% fall in the FEV_1 is more than $8\,\mu$mol ($16\,$mg/ml), the abnormality can be regarded as minimal.

DIAGNOSIS

In most patients the disease can be diagnosed from the history. Asthma typically causes episodes of wheezing, chest tightness, or

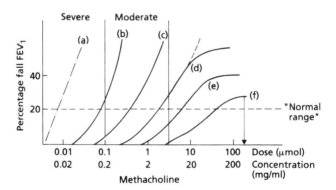

Figure 3-1. Dose/concentration response curves to methacholine showing different degrees of airway hyperresponsiveness, typical of a patient with severe asthma (A), with moderate asthma (B and C), and mild asthma (D and E). The normal range is indicated in (F). The tests are usually terminated when a dose of 4.0 μmol has been given, but the full curves can be described using higher doses. Similar curves are seen in response to histamine. Reprinted from Busse WW, Holgate ST. Asthma and Rhinitis. Boston: Blackwell Science, 1995.

cough which remit spontaneously or in response to a bronchodilator, but the onset of symptoms of breathlessness can be insidious.

Consideration must be given to an alternative diagnosis in some patients. These include older patients who have smoked and may have chronic obstructive pulmonary disease; infants below three years who may have bronchiolitis; children with frequent chest infections, who may have cystic fibrosis; severe airways obstruction and dyspnea in a young person, who may have bronchiolitis obliterans; and patients who have episodes of unexplained breathlessness and may have hyperventilation, vocal cord dysfunction, or panic attacks. If the management plan outlined below is followed, the diagnosis as well as the form and severity of the asthma soon becomes apparent.

MANAGEMENT PLAN
Reasons for management plan

The multiplicity of drugs available to treat asthma in recent years has caused confusion to both patients and physicians. Which drugs should be used by which patient and for how long? This problem, coupled with the fact that asthma mortality has been increasing in some populations, has led to the writing of guidelines for the management of asthma. Although these plans differ in the approach to the patient, their aims are similar. They are "best guesses" at a logical approach because there are no long-term controlled trials of different forms of treatment in well-defined groups of patients. In addition, there are no data available to predict if, in the long term, the complications of the disease are decreased by the use of management plans.

The management plan described here and outlined in Table 3-1 is a way of describing the steps that are necessary for the complete care of the individual patient. It emphasizes assessment of the patient so that the best treatment can be introduced from the beginning. The steps are not necessarily carried out in the order in which they are presented. Most asthmatics who present to respiratory physicians have severe or complicated disease, and it takes a long time to gain control of the disease and for the patient to be able to undertake the greater part of his or her own management. In addition, the concept of caring for the patient for a long time, perhaps for life, is a recent feature of treatment and an important one for children as well as for adults.

Phase 1—assessment	Phase 2—treatment	Phase 3—commitment
1. Form & severity	1. Drugs for asthma	1. Action plan for deterioration
2. Causal & provoking factors	2. Drugs for symptoms	2. Education
3. Aggravating factors	3. Allergen avoidance	3. Regular review
4. Reversibility ("usual best" PEF)	4. Hyposensitization	
5. Complications	5. Miscellaneous	

Table 3-1.   Management Plan

Phase 1—assessment

Each patient with symptoms that suggest asthma needs a complete assessment of the disease, including its form and severity, its likely causes, the present provoking and aggravating factors, the degree of reversibility of lung function, and the potential complications. Appropriate treatment can then be introduced.

Form and severity: Using the history and simple tests of lung function, the form (episodic, persistent) and severity (severe, moderate, mild) can be determined in most patients in a few days. Some of the features of the different forms and severity of the disease are shown in Table 3-2. The variability of peak flow readings (PEFvar) is calculated from morning and evening recordings over seven to ten days (as shown in Figure 3-2), at a time when the patient is not having an acute exacerbation. It is the range of values in a given day divided by the highest. The mean variability over a week or more is then used in assessing severity. If wished, a combined score out of 12 with 0 to 4 for symptoms, 0 to 4 for bronchodilator use, and 0 to 4 for PEFvar can be made. A patient with a score of less than 6 has mild disease, 6 to 8 is moderate, and more than 8 is severe.

The measurement of AHR, using a dose or concentration response curve to histamine or methacholine, and expressed as PD_{20} or PC_{20} values, is of added help in some patients. In cross-sectional studies, PEFvar correlates well with measurements of AHR, although the correlation is not as good in the individual with time, and the correlation of both AHR and PEFvar with symptoms is not consistent, probably because each measures a different aspect of airway function.

Table 3-2. Classification of Asthma Severity[a]

Severity of asthma	Clinical features before treatment	Lung function	Regular medication usually required to maintain control
Mild	Intermittent, brief symptoms <1–2 times a week Nocturnal asthma symptoms <2 times a month Asymptomatic between exacerbations	PEF >80% predicted at baseline PEF variability <20% PEF normal after bronchodilator	Intermittent inhaled short-acting β-agonist (taken as needed) only
Moderate	Exacerbations >1–2 times a week Nocturnal asthma symptoms >2 times a month Symptoms requiring inhaled β-agonist almost daily	PEF 60–80% predicted at baseline PEF variability 20–30% PEF normal after bronchodilator	Daily inhaled anti-inflammatory agent Possibly a daily long-acting bronchodilator, especially for nocturnal symptoms
Severe	Frequent exacerbations Continuous symptoms Frequent nocturnal asthma symptoms Physical activities limited by asthma Hospitalization for asthma in previous year[b] Previous life-threatening exacerbation[b]	PEF <60% predicted at baseline PEF variability >30% PEF below normal despite optimal therapy	Daily inhaled anti-inflammatory agent at high doses Daily long-acting bronchodilator, especially for nocturnal symptoms Frequent use of systemic corticosteroids

[a]Note: The characteristics noted in this table are general, and the characteristics may overlap because asthma is highly variable. Furthermore, a patient's classification may change over time. One or more features may be present to be assigned a grade of severity; a patient should usually be assigned to the most severe grade in which any feature occurs. Once the minimum medication required to maintain control of asthma has been identified, then this medication requirement reflects the overall severity of the condition.

[b]The potential severity—related to a patient's past history (for example, a previous life-threatening exacerbation or a hospitalization for asthma in the previous year) as well as present status—should be considered at all times.

Source: International Consensus Report on Diagnosis and Treatment of Asthma. National Heart, Lung and Blood Institute, National Institutes of Health, Bethesda, MD, 1992 (Clin Exp Allergy 1992;22[suppl 1]).

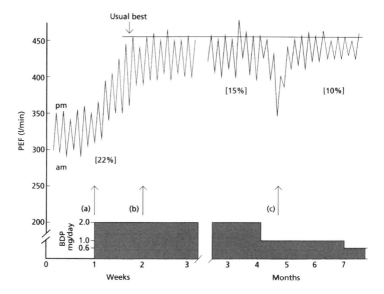

Figure 3-2. The peak expiratory flow rates of a 40-year-old woman of 160 cm (predicted = 480 L per minute) over a period of seven months. Daily readings and then weekly readings are shown. The lines connect values recorded in the morning on waking (A.M.) and in the evening before bed (P.M.). Oral corticosteroids (50 mg/day) were started at point A and stopped at point B when there was no further improvement in the A.M. readings. The "usual best" value is indicated. At point C an exacerbation occurred and was treated for four days with additional oral corticosteroids. The mean variability (range divided by highest) for a week at the beginning [20%] decreases to 15% at three months and to 10% by six months. The doses of inhaled beclomethasone dipropionate (BDP) prescribed are shown. Reprinted from Busse WW, Holgate ST. Asthma and Rhinitis. Boston: Blackwell Science, 1995.

Tests of responsiveness are safe and can be performed in the clinic in a few minutes using histamine or methacholine. The full curves shown in Figure 3-1 are usually not constructed, and the dose is stopped at 8 µmol or after the FEV_1 has fallen by 20%. Provided that the patient has near-normal lung function, is not recovering from a recent exacerbation, and has not taken inhaled bronchodilator drugs for six hours, values for PD_{20} FEV_1 of less than 4.0 µmol indicate an abnormality that is likely to be associated with symptoms. Values below 0.1 µmol indicate severe asthma and an increased likelihood of life-threatening attack. On the other hand, a completely normal curve makes it unlikely that the airway has developed the changes seen in persistent asthma. Once a baseline value for the degree of responsiveness has been established, it can be regarded as a reliable guide to the severity of the underlying airway problem and used as a baseline for following the progress of the disease. It is also useful in patient education.

Other tests of respiratory function are used in the assessment of the severity of disease in patients with asthma. If the spirometric function is abnormal, treatment to establish the best value (see below) is indicated. Unless already in treatment, patients with severe disease usually have some degree of airflow limitation and of hyperinflation. If there has been prolonged hyperinflation of the lungs in childhood, there is likely to be loss of elastic recoil, probably caused by enlarged air spaces. In patients with asthma who have never smoked, the diffusing capacity is usually normal and is a useful test for distinguishing asthma from emphysema.

Causal and provoking factors: The factors that may have induced the disease or are acting as continuing sources of provocation must be defined. There is good evidence that allergens, particularly from house dust mites, cats, and *Alternaria*, cause asthma and, based on the occupational model, it is unlikely that complete control of the disease can occur while the patient remains exposed to these allergens.

The patient may not have identified all the important provoking agents, especially those at the workplace, if the agents cause late responses and the symptoms occur mainly at night. Some allergens, and importantly mites, rarely cause episodes of airway narrowing, and the patient may be unaware of being allergic so that the allergic status must be documented objectively. This is done simply and quickly with skin prick tests using common airborne allergens. It is necessary to include two or three allergens from each of four groups (mites and cockroaches, animals, pollens, and molds). Cross-reactivity to allergens within these groups means that it is not necessary to test large numbers of individual allergens. If all are negative it is unlikely that the patient is allergic to an important airborne allergen. Skin tests are done not in order to desensitize the patient but to make the patient aware of the relevant allergens so that steps can be taken to decrease the levels of exposure.

Ingested substances that cause acute attacks, such as aspirin, some foods, and drinks that contain metabisulfite, are usually recognized by the patient, but if doubt exists, a specific challenge test with the food or with metabisulfite can be performed. The role of exercise in inducing attacks can be documented with a standard exercise test and repeated after appropriate aerosol treatment to determine the best drug or combination of drugs that prevent the airway narrowing. If an occupational agent is suspected, a careful history plus challenges with one or more of the putative agents used at the workplace may be required.

Aggravating factors: Of the factors that appear to aggravate asthma, rhinitis is the most important. Although it is difficult to show that treatment of rhinitis improves the control of asthma, there is evidence that rhinitis precipitates attacks, and there is no doubt that a clear nasal airway improves the quality of life and the quality of sleep.

Gastroesophageal reflux appears to be an aggravating factor in some patients, and patients who are taking theophylline often complain of heartburn. Treatment with an appropriate drug to decrease acid secretion often improves the control of symptoms and the patient's quality of life. Obstruction of the upper airway during sleep is another aggravating factor, and excessive daytime sleepiness, dry mouth on waking, and evidence of noisy breathing during sleep should be asked about, a sleep study should be performed, and, if necessary, the obstruction should be treated.

Reversibility of peak expiratory flow rates—concept of "usual best": The peak flow rate is a simple, practical guide to the state of the airways at any given time. It can be used to determine the reversibility of airway narrowing, as a guide to severity, and to indicate the level of control of the disease at a given point in time. Figure 3-2 shows recordings of peak flow rate in a patient at the beginning of treatment and during a course of oral corticosteroids.

If the peak flow reading is close to the predicted value when the patient is first seen, this value can be used as the "usual best" and forms the basis for writing action plans (below) and for adjusting the dose of inhaled corticosteroids. If it is less than 90% of the predicted value after a β-agonist is inhaled, the degree of reversibility is best documented by giving a short course of oral corticosteroids (for ten days or less if maximal improvement is achieved). The corticosteroid is given either in divided doses or in the late afternoon in daily doses of about 1.0 mg/kg body weight. The corticosteroid is then stopped, without stepwise decreases, and the inhaled corticosteroids are continued. The peak flow readings during this time are carefully documented before and after doses of bronchodilator aerosols. This allows the calculation of variability and the documentation of the "usual best," which is the best value obtained on several occasions over a few days. The "usual best" is one of the values on which daily drug therapy is based. Some physicians prefer to introduce or increase the dose of inhaled corticosteroids (ICS) rather than use oral steroids to define the reversibility and the "usual best" value. The "usual best" value often increases with time, in children with growth or in adults as the airway wall inflammation gradually improves.

Complications: Apart from the complications of severe acute attacks and irreversible airflow limitation, the important complications of asthma in adults are bronchopulmonary aspergillosis (described below), mucoid impaction, and bronchiectasis. These are assessed from the history and appropriate immunological tests. Bronchiectasis can be documented with a CAT scan if it is thought that an intervention might be necessary. The potential complications (hypertension, diabetes, osteoporosis, cataracts) of corticosteroid therapy should be assessed in patients taking regular doses of these drugs.

Phase 2—treatment

Drugs for asthma: The aim of using drugs is to decrease the long-term effects of airway inflammation. The drugs known to do this are the corticosteroids and, to a lesser extent, the cromones. The drugs and their doses depend on the form and severity of the disease, the age of the patient, and increasingly, the ability of the patient to afford them. The drugs themselves are described in the following sections. The guidelines in Figure 3-3 for their use in the management plan are helpful.

1. The cromones (sodium cromoglycate and nedocromil sodium) help to prevent symptoms when given before known provoking factors such as exercise; they help to control the symptoms of seasonal asthma, and they are useful in controlling mild disease, but they do little to change the severity of persistent disease.
2. The cromones are extremely safe and virtually without long-term side effects. To be effective in long-term control, they must be used in adequate doses and at least three to four times a day.

3. The more severe the disease, the less it is possible to decrease the severity, as judged by symptoms, PEFvar, and AHR, to a clinically important extent, by any means other than inhaled corticosteroids and allergen avoidance.

4. The more severe the disease, the higher the dose of inhaled corticosteroid needed, and the higher the dose, the quicker the response. The response can be expected within days in relation to symptoms and within weeks for changes in AHR or PEFvar.

5. Doses of ICS (see Figure 3-3) should be used for an initial period of three to six months and then reduced to a level that prevents exacerbations. With the correct dose, improvement may continue for many months, and it is important that the patient knows that complete control may take a long time.

6. The doses of ICS used depend on severity (see Figure 3-3). They should be used for three to six months, and the severity reassessed and the doses adjusted. The symptoms improve within days, and changes in PEFvar took place within weeks. Some maintenance ICS is needed once the disease is controlled. *In practice, most patients stop taking ICS when their symptoms improve and start them again when the symptoms reappear.*

7. The usual best peak flow rate is a useful value against which to titrate the drugs in most patients. However, some patients use the early morning value and others use symptoms. In practice, a mixture of symptoms, bronchodilator use, and PEFvar, as shown in Table 3-2 and Figure 3-3, is the best guide.

8. Oral corticosteroids should be used to find the usual best PEF, for exacerbations (see below), and in a few patients whose disease is not controlled by the inhaled forms. The lowest dose possible is indicated because of the long-term side effects. The drugs are most effective when given at 3 P.M.

Drugs for symptoms: It is not possible to describe all the drugs used to relieve symptoms. The following guidelines are helpful.

1. Most patients need some form of bronchodilator therapy, and β-agonist aerosols are the most effective. They are prescribed for symptoms or if the PEF is below a set level (e.g., 60% of the usual best). Patients with severe disease may need β-agonist aerosols frequently until the airway inflammation improves.

2. High doses of β-agonist drugs, taken as aerosols on a regular basis, may make asthma worse. The evidence for this is discussed

Step-up: Progression to the next higher step is indicated when control cannot be achieved at the current step and there is assurance that medication is used correctly. If PEFR ≤60% predicted or personal best, consider a burst of oral corticosteroids and then proceed.

Step-down: Reduction in therapy is considered when the outcome for therapy has been achieved and sustained for several weeks or even months at the current step. Reduction in therapy is also needed to identify the minimum therapy required to maintain control.

Outcome: Control of Asthma
- Minimal (ideally no) chronic symptoms, including nocturnal symptoms
- Minimal (infrequent) episodes
- No emergency visits
- Minimal need for p.r.n. β_2-agonist
- No limitations on activities, including exercise
- PEF circadian variation <20%
- (Near) normal PEF
- Minimal (or no) adverse effects from medicine

Outcome: Best Possible Results
- Fewest symptoms
- Least need for p.r.n. β_2-agonist
- Least limitation of activity
- Least PEFR circadian variation
- Best PEFR
- Fewest adverse effects from medicine

Therapy*
- Inhaled corticosteroid 800–1000µg daily (>1000µg under specialist's supervision) and
- Sustained release theophylline and/or

Therapy*
- Inhaled corticosteroids daily 800–1000µg

Therapy*
- Inhaled anti-inflammatory daily

Step-Down
- Once control is reached at

Therapy* • Short acting inhaled β_2-agonist p.r.n. not more than 3× a week • Short acting inhaled β_2-agonist or cromolyn before exercise or exposure to antigen	initially: Inhaled corticosteroid 200–500µg or cromolyn or nedocromil (children begin with a trial of cromolyn) – If necessary: inhaled corticosteroid 400–750µg (alternatively, particularly for nocturnal symptoms, proceed to Step 3 with additional long acting bronchodilator) and • Short acting inhaled β_2-agonist p.r.n., not to exceed 3–4 times a day	(> 1000µg under specialist's supervision) and • Sustained release theophylline, oral β_2-agonist, or long acting inhaled β_2-agonist, especially for nocturnal symptoms; may consider inhaled anticholinergics and • Short acting inhaled β_2-agonist p.r.n., not to exceed 3–4 times a day	oral β_2 agonist, or long acting inhaled β_2-agonist, especially for nocturnal symptoms with or without • Short acting inhaled β_2-agonist once a day; may consider inhaled anticholinergic and • Oral corticosteroids (alternate day or single daily dose) and • Short acting inhaled β_2-agonist p.r.n., up to 3–4 times a day	any step, and sustained, a step down reduction in therapy may be carefully considered and is needed to identify the minimum therapy required to maintain control.
Clinical Features Pretreatment[†] • Intermittent, brief symptoms <1–2× a week • Nocturnal asthma symptoms <1–2× a month • Asymptomatic between exacerbations • PEFR or FEV_1 – >80% predicted – variability <20%	Clinical Features Pretreatment[†] • Exacerbations >1–2×a week • Exacerbations may affect activity and sleep • Nocturnal asthma symptoms >2× a month • Chronic symptoms requiring short acting β_2-agonist almost daily • PEFR or FEV_1 – 60–80% predicted – variability 20–30%		Clinical Features Pretreatment[†] • Frequent exacerbations • Continuous symptoms • Frequent nocturnal asthma symptoms • Physical activities limited by asthma • PEFR or FEV_1 – <60% predicted – variability >30%	• Advise patients of signs of worsening asthma and actions to control it.
Step 1: Mild	Step 2: Moderate	Step 3: Moderate	Step 4: Severe	

* All therapy must include patient education about prevention (including environmental control where appropriate) as well as control of symptoms.
[†] One or more features may be present to be assigned a grade of severity; an individual should usually be assigned to the most severe grade in which any feature occurs. Source: International Consensus Report on the Diagnosis and Treatment of Asthma. National Heart, Lung and Blood Institute, National Institutes of Health, Bethesda, MD 1992 (Clin Exp Allergy 1992;22[suppl 1]).

Figure 3-3. Chronic management of asthma: stepwise approach to asthma therapy

below. Patients should be reassured that the drugs are safe for acute attacks but are not indicated for the treatment of the disease. If possible, they should not be used on a regular basis.

3. Some patients have severe symptoms that are not controlled by inhaled drugs. Some need regular theophylline. When theophylline is being used in conjunction with β-agonist aerosols for symptoms, the dose can be found by trial and error.

4. Anticholinergics have a small place as acute bronchodilators for attacks and more regularly in older patients with obstructed airways.

Allergen avoidance: The occupational model strongly suggests that continuing exposure to an allergen is associated with ongoing or deteriorating disease in spite of treatment, and it is known that allergen avoidance can decrease the severity of asthma. Since in most populations house dust mites have been found to be the dominant allergen, it makes sense to reduce the domestic levels of these allergens. Lowering allergen levels takes considerable effort, but it can be done. In addition, it is possible to remove cat and dog allergens. The situation with mold allergen is less clear but, by decreasing indoor humidity through increasing the ventilation in houses, it may be possible to reduce the amount of domestic mold allergen.

Immunotherapy: Allergists have used immunotherapy injections to treat patients with asthma for many years, and there is some evidence that some patients are improved by this treatment. However, even in placebo-controlled trials, the long-term outcomes are not stated, the duration of improvement is rarely evaluated, and the changes in AHR, as measured by challenges with histamine and methacholine, have rarely been studied. It may well become the treatment of choice if a method can be found to control T-cell function, but at present it should be used only as an adjunct to appropriate pharmacological treatment for patients with asthma.

Phase 3—commitment

A long-term plan, worked out by the physician and the patient together, is needed. This plan should include a written action plan for exacerbations, guidelines by which the doses of drugs are to be adjusted, education of the patient and family about the disease, and regular review.

Action plan for deteriorating asthma: Any patient who has persistent asthma needs a written plan with instructions about the action to take if his or her asthma deteriorates either slowly or rapidly. This requires that the usual best and usual morning peak flow rates are known, as well as the expected response to a bronchodilator aerosol when the reading is low. Peak flow readings on waking that are gradually getting worse or increasing variability of flow rates over several days indicate deterioration requiring either an increased dose of ICS or the introduction of oral corticosteroids. In some patients symptoms change before the PEF falls, and such patients should be alerted to alter the dose of ICS when these changed symptoms occur. In general, experience shows that a course of prednisone (1.0 mg per kg per day) for a short time is effective. Instructions about doses and when and how to increase and decrease them again should be written down on the daily diary card.

Education: It is well recognized that the control of asthma improves with education that is aimed at self-management, and in many centers asthma education clinics have been established, similar to those already established for helping diabetic patients. The success of such clinics is difficult to evaluate unless all other factors are kept constant, but they appear to have improved the quality of life of many patients.

Regular review: Patients with persistent asthma have an incurable disease and thus need continuing care. This concept is rarely discussed because there is always an element of hope that the disease will disappear. Obviously it is important to sustain this hope and give long-term support. Physicians should stay in contact with their patients and review the doses of drugs with time, ensure that lung function is not deteriorating more rapidly than expected, and ensure that peak flow monitoring is continued where necessary and that provoking stimuli are being avoided. Families of patients need to know that the children of allergic parents are likely to be allergic and that avoiding exposure to house dust mite allergen during infancy should be a priority.

DRUGS USED IN THE TREATMENT OF ASTHMA
Inhaled corticosteroids

Clinical effects: Corticosteroids are the most effective class of drugs for the treatment of asthma, and the development of inhaled forms is the greatest single advance in asthma treatment in the last 20 years. Their effectiveness probably rests on their multiplicity of action, particularly in reducing the number of cytokines and therefore the number of inflammatory cells, particularly eosinophils, in the airway walls. It is stressed that ICS, although acting like other steroids within cells, are important because they affect cells in the lumen. In usual doses, ICS have an effect on AHR that is not seen with doses of prednisone that can be used in the long term, and patients who were poorly controlled on high doses of oral steroids 20 years ago improved greatly with the introduction of ICS.

It is now documented by a large number of studies that ICS improve the severity of asthma in most patients as judged by levels of AHR, and they are more effective than β-agonists or theophylline in controlling the disease. Studies of the effects of ICS on AHR clearly show that no other drugs, except unacceptably high doses of prednisone, can reduce the severity of asthma.

Precise use: In spite of the large number of studies, the dose of ICS required in the individual patient is not well established. In general, in moderately severe disease the starting dose is 1 mg and for severe disease 2 mg per day in divided doses, but these doses may change as newer, more potent preparations become available. It is necessary to have a goal for the outcome of therapy in each patient, and it is the achievement of this outcome, rather than a fixed dose schedule, that is important. Thus, once the patient has moved from the category of severe to that of moderate asthma, the dose can be decreased, but it must be appreciated that improvement continues for many months and sometimes years. It does not seem possible to stop ICS completely in patients who have been documented as having severe asthma. Many patients do stop taking them, but eventually the symptoms reappear, although apparent control may last for weeks or even months. The maintenance dose needed is usually found by trial and error. There is some evidence that nedocromil sodium allows the dose to be decreased.

At the practical level, when a metered-dose aerosol is used, it is important to use a spacing device. This appears to minimize the local and systemic effects and to lower the dose needed to achieve or maintain control. A spacing device does not appear to be needed with the dry powder forms of the drugs.

There are some patients who fail to respond to high doses of ICS. Rather than continue with high doses, steps need to be taken to define the causes of this failure. These are outlined below under "steroid resistant asthma." However, in the great majority of patients, with adherence to a management plan, it is possible to reduce the severity of asthma and to maintain the control using a regular maintenance dose. If the plan is successful, no other drug therapy is needed.

Compliance: This is a major problem in long-term treatment. Because ICS do not have any acute effect on symptoms, because the patient knows that steroids cause side effects, and because they are expensive in most communities, patients often forget or neglect to take the prescribed doses. Compliance can be improved by giving the drug twice daily, by using the high-dose forms of the inhalers, by minimizing side effects, and by a continuing education program.

Side effects: Candidiasis of the throat and dysphonia are local side effects of these drugs. Candidiasis is usually not a problem because it can be treated with local antifungal agents without stopping the asthma drug and can be reduced by using a spacer with the aerosol and by gargling after each administration. Dysphonia, which is not related to the candidiasis and may be a myopathy of the laryngeal muscles, may be more difficult to avoid.

Adrenal suppression is found most in those who take high doses. The degree of suppression is not usually severe enough to cause concern itself, but it is a marker of a systemic effect. Clinical evidence of excessive steroid use, including bruising, weight gain, and possibly osteoporosis, can be found in patients who take high doses of these drugs. Concerns about bone growth in children are commonly expressed, but it appears that children with severe asthma who need ICS to control the disease attain their expected height, albeit somewhat later than their nonasthmatic peers.

Some physicians have expressed concern that responses to ICS may decrease with time, but this has not been evaluated objectively. It is possible that this occurs, and a short period without the drugs may restore the responsiveness. If this is the case then intermittent therapy, which is practiced by the great majority of patients in real life, might come to be viewed as the best method of administering these drugs.

All corticosteroids are potentially harmful, and ICS should be given in doses that are appropriate to the current severity of the disease. There are no studies in which doses above 2 mg/day have been shown to lessen the severity of disease when lower doses have failed, so the dose should not be increased indefinitely.

Cost effectiveness: At present, these drugs are now affordable in many nonaffluent populations. Although there have been no formal publications about their cost effectiveness, it is likely that they could be shown to be extremely cost-effective because, once asthma is controlled, most patients with persistent disease can be maintained on a small dose without any other drug. However, gaining good control in someone with severe disease takes time and needs constant attention to the details of the management plan.

Cromones

The drugs sodium cromoglycate (SCG) and nedocromil sodium (NS) are collectively called cromones. Although they have a somewhat different range of actions, they are discussed together.

Clinical effects: Their main action is to prevent the early and late responses to inhaled allergens and the responses to a number of indirect stimuli that cause attacks of asthma. When administered before challenges, SCG and NS inhibit or greatly modify the response to exercise, nebulized water, allergens, hyperventilation with cold air, sulfur dioxide, adenosine, and bradykinin. It appears that NS is slightly more potent than SCG in protecting against provoked attacks.

Since there is evidence that repeated allergen challenges involving late asthmatic responses make asthma worse, it would be expected that these drugs would markedly improve asthma. When SCG was first available, it made a big difference to the lives of many patients because it had no side effects, prevented attacks, and was used to control the disease in many patients with mild disease. In patients with persistent disease it has proved to be less effective than ICS and thus, in the last few years, it has been used less frequently in adults. However, the high doses of ICS used by some patients are causing worry about known and possibly unrecognized long-term effects, and NS can be used to decrease the dose of ICS needed to maintain control.

After 30 years of use and investigation with SCG and several years with NS, their modes of action are still not known. It seems likely that SCG has several actions, including protecting the sensory nerve endings, a small effect in limiting degranulation of mast cells, and an effect on IgE production, and both have an effect on eosinophils, which may be greater for NS than SCG. There is evidence that NS may be a more potent mast cell stabilizer than SCG.

In the management plan, they are used to prevent the effects of provoking stimuli and to control the disease when it is mild. There is evidence from trials that they decrease the degree of AHR in many patients but, in comparison with corticosteroids, they do little to improve airway function in patients with persistent disease. Cromoglycate is effective in patients with episodic disease and modifies AHR in patients with pollen-induced asthma if taken during the season.

The choice of drug will depend on local circumstances. At present SCG is used mostly in children, although it is effective in adults, while NS has been introduced for the treatment of adults, where it may have some steroid-sparing effects.

Methods of administration: These drugs are administered by the inhalation route. Originally, as a dry powder, 20 mg of SCG was inhaled from a Spinhaler. Both drugs are now available in metered-dose form, which allows greater penetration into the lungs and makes SCG effective at a lower dose. In trials, SCG has been shown to be effective in patients of all ages and with different forms of asthma, but clinical experience suggests that it is most effective in young patients with mild to moderately severe asthma. Many children can be maintained on this drug alone, but it must be used in adequate doses (5 mg from a metered-dose inhaler) and three to four times a day for a period of weeks to gain the benefit of prolonged inhibition of mediator release in the airways.

Side effects: These drugs are safe, with a very low rate of side effects. In the spincap form some patients complain of throat irritation, but this is not a problem with the aerosol form. Some patients complain of the taste of these drugs.

Cost-effectiveness: In countries that do not have a health service that provides drugs free of charge, these drugs are too expensive for the majority of patients. In patients with mild disease, there is evidence that SCG is cost-effective by reducing the number of hospital visits. Their lack of long-term side effects, rather than their cost effectiveness, is the factor most likely to determine their place in therapy in coming years.

β-agonists

Modes of action: The effectiveness of β-adrenoceptor agonist drugs in both treating and preventing asthma attacks has led to their widespread use and to a large number of studies relating to their modes of action. They relax contracted smooth muscle, prevent contraction of the smooth muscle by various stimuli in a dose-related manner, increase mucociliary clearance, decrease the release of mediators from cells near the epithelial surface, and protect against leakage from postcapillary venules.

Method of administration: Inhalation is the chosen method of administration of β-agonists because this route allows a lower dose and fewer side effects as well as good protective action against provoked attacks. Inhaled β-agonists have been shown to protect (usually in a dose-related manner) against many forms of provocation including allergens, exercise, osmotic stimuli, histamine, methacholine, and sulfur dioxide. The mechanism of this protective action is not understood, although it is known that it is not due simply to relaxation of the smooth muscle.

β-agonists are available orally and for injection, but tremor and palpitations are usually more marked with systemic administration. The exception is the systemic administration of sustained-release forms for treatment of nocturnal asthma. For the very young and the elderly, who may have difficulty with metered aerosols, a number of methods are available for the administration of aerosols, including spacers, rotacaps, and nebulizers. These alternative methods should be explored if the advantages of the inhaled route are to be maximized.

Side effects: In the acute situation, these drugs appear to be safe although they cause the predictable side effects of palpitations and tremor, especially in patients who use them intermittently in high doses. These effects are rarely complained of by patients who use them regularly in moderate doses. Interestingly, the airways of asthmatic patients do not become tolerant to them.

Safety: Recently there has been discussion about the long-term safety of these drugs. The problem was first raised in relation to fenoterol, which was commonly used regularly and in high doses in New Zealand. A series of case-control studies strongly implicates fenoterol; however, the severity of asthma in these patients remains a problem in interpreting the degree to which fenoterol accounted for the epidemic of deaths that occurred in that country. It is possible that the β-agonists used in high doses on a regular basis make asthma worse in some individuals, and the regular use of isoproterenol may have been the cause of the epidemic of deaths which occurred in some countries in the 1960s. Inhalation of fenoterol on a regular basis has been shown to cause lung function to deteriorate, AHR to increase, and the control of asthma to deteriorate. More recent evidence suggests that regular, daily use of albuterol (2 puffs q.i.d.) in mild asthmatics is not associated with a deterioration of asthma control nor increases in AHR. However, it appears that ordinary doses of albuterol and terbutaline do not alter the severity of asthma in most patients.

Long-acting forms: Long-acting forms of β-agonist drugs (e.g., salmeterol) have been available for several years. They were developed at a time when the usefulness of β-agonists in preventing attacks had been acknowledged and few questions were being asked about their long-term effects. These drugs have proved to be effective at both bronchodilating and protecting against provoked attacks. However, their place in long-term treatment is not yet known because, with better forms of ICS and the emphasis on controlling inflammation, there seems little place for them except in patients with severe disease. It will be important to establish whether there is a subgroup of patients whose asthma is worsened by β-agonists before clinicians will feel comfortable prescribing these drugs to patients other than those with severe disease.

Cost effectiveness: The short-acting (6–8 hour) β-agonists are now cheap enough to be afforded by most people of the world and they are probably cost-effective for symptomatic relief. It is too early to determine the cost effectiveness of the newly available long-acting (12-hour) β-agonists.

Oral corticosteroids

Clinical effects: These drugs are not the treatment of choice for the long-term control of patients with asthma, and their use, wherever possible, should be confined to pulses of drug to prevent or treat exacerbations. For this reason they are discussed separately from the inhaled forms. They are especially useful during severe attacks that do not respond to β-agonists.

Mode of delivery: There is evidence that these drugs are best given at 3 P.M., when they will be most effective in dealing with nocturnal symptoms. In severe attacks they are usually given more frequently. If low doses are needed on a long-term basis, they should be used on alternate days if possible.

49

Side effects: Short-term use of these drugs even in high doses is associated with few side effects. Occasionally, psychiatric disturbance occurs, and some patients complain of blurred vision, which reverses on lowering the dose.

The side effects of oral corticosteroids taken for prolonged periods have been known for many years. In particular, the effects on the bones in adults (osteoporosis) may be more serious than the underlying asthma. Suppression of the normal adrenal production of cortisol occurs after 10 to 14 days of treatment, and much attention has been given to this effect because it can be measured easily. However, it is probably of importance only in patients being weaned from long-term oral doses, who must be warned that they are at risk if they sustain major trauma or surgery. It is the effects on blood pressure (blood glucose), appearance, bones, and eyes (cataracts) that are serious and mean that these drugs must be avoided if possible. Fortunately, the inhaled forms allow this to be done in most patients, and the oral forms can be used as pulse treatment for exacerbations.

Cost effectiveness: Prednisone tablets are cheap and easier to take than inhaled drugs. For these two reasons large numbers of asthmatic patients continue to take them. This may prove cost-effective in the long term for patients who can be controlled on low doses, but for doses above 10 mg per day the side effects, which often lead to the need for other drugs (such as antihypertensives) and to further disability, may make them less cost-effective than the aerosol forms.

Theophylline

Clinical effects: The methylxanthines, in particular theophylline, are effective bronchodilators when adequate serum concentrations are maintained, although the way in which theophylline produces a therapeutic effect is unknown. In addition to its bronchodilating actions, it may have some anti-inflammatory effects because it decreases the release of mediators from mast cells and reduces microvascular permeability. Its role as a prophylactic drug is unclear. Compared with β-agonist aerosols, theophylline has only small effects on exercise-induced asthma and on methacholine- and histamine-induced asthma. In the long term it has no effect on the degree of AHR.

Clinical use: The clinical use of theophylline varies greatly among countries. In general, it is more widely used in countries where β$_2$-

agonist aerosols are infrequently used. The drug must be given with care to achieve adequate, but not toxic, serum levels. The slow-release forms of the drug allow this to be achieved, and the number of patients experiencing side effects has decreased. The main uses of the drug are in the treatment of a subgroup of patients with severe asthma and who have more symptoms without it. The mode of action in these patients is unknown. In patients with severe airways obstruction, particularly those with chronic obstructive pulmonary disease (COPD), it is sometimes useful in controlling symptoms that may be related to its ability to increase the contractility of the diaphragm.

Side effects: The side effects are well known and are related to the plasma concentrations of the drug. It causes nausea, vomiting, headache, and restlessness. At high concentrations, it can cause cardiac arrhythmias and occasionally convulsions. Concern has been expressed about behavioral disturbances in children but the overall importance of this is hard to establish. If the dose of theophylline is high enough to disturb sleep, it may have an indirect effect on daytime behavior. Some adult patients find theophylline beneficial, while others cannot tolerate it, especially if their asthma has been well controlled with other drugs.

Other bronchodilating drugs

The synthetic anticholinergic drugs ipratropium bromide and oxitropium bromide are widely used as bronchodilators. They have anticholinergic activity but do not have the side effects of atropine derivatives because they are poorly absorbed systemically. Ipratropium has been used for almost 20 years and is more effective as a bronchodilator for daily use than the β-agonists although it may have an additive effect in some patients. Without a trial, there appears to be no way of predicting which patients will benefit from the drug. They are delivered as aerosols and have few side effects. There is no evidence that they cause drying of secretions.

SPECIAL TREATMENT PROBLEMS
Steroid-resistant asthma

As inhaled corticosteroids are increasingly used, most clinicians find that most patients improve, so that when a patient fails to respond or appears to need very high doses, the term *steroid-resistant asthma*

(SRA) is used. It occurs in a small number of patients, but these patients use a disproportionate amount of resources.

Before a label of SRA is given, the following criteria should be satisfied: First, it should be demonstrated that the patient has asthma, because sometimes one may be misdiagnosed, as discussed above. To be really sure, a bronchial biopsy may be necessary, because the disease has a typical histological appearance. Second, the patient must take adequate amounts of ICS in a form that ensures that the drug reaches the airway (dry powder, aerosol with a spacer, or a nebulized form and at least 2.0 mg/day). Third, all provoking stimuli, especially domestic allergens, must be removed. Fourth, all potential aggravating factors must be investigated and treated, including gastroesophageal reflux, rhinitis, and obstructed breathing during sleep. Finally, use of β-agonists must be changed from regular use to occasional doses for severe symptoms. After these criteria are met, the patient should then be managed with a strict plan for at least six months. Failure to respond can only then be designated as SRA.

Failure of the lung function to return to normal after treatment for ten days with oral steroid, in a patient with previously documented asthma and good lung function, is classified as SRA for research studies, but in clinical practice the label SRA can be applied only after the measures outlined above have been undertaken. Abnormal lung function in an asthmatic by itself does not mean SRA if the symptoms are well controlled by ICS.

Once the diagnosis is established, other anti-inflammatory drugs including methotrexate, cyclosporin, or gold can be tried. However, these drugs are toxic, and methotrexate is not uniformly effective and has even been a cause of asthma. For these reasons, and because ICS are so effective, these toxic drugs should be given only when there is good evidence of resistance to the action of ICS.

A number of theories for steroid resistance have been put forward. The abnormality appears to be a general defect in the ability of all cells to respond to glucocorticoids. This inability may be inherent or acquired.

Asthma in pregnancy

There is evidence that a low FEV_1 during pregnancy leads to retardation of intrauterine growth, although not necessarily to prematurity. This means that during pregnancy the FEV_1 should be maintained at the best possible value with the available drugs.

There is little evidence that any of the drugs discussed above (albuterol, beclomethasone, theophylline, and cromones) have any harmful effects on the fetus. In particular, inhaled corticosteroids (beclomethasone) appear to have no harmful effect on fetal development and should be given to keep the asthma well controlled.

Nocturnal symptoms of asthma

There is no evidence that people who have symptoms of wheezing at night have a special kind of asthma, but these symptoms indicate that the airway abnormality is severe or that the patient is exposed to a substance during the day that is causing late asthmatic responses. Many things combine to make airway narrowing worse at night. These include a decrease in circulating adrenaline and cortisol, the supine posture, snoring, exposure to house dust mite allergen in the bedding, late asthmatic responses to allergens inhaled during the day, and gastroesophageal reflux. There is good evidence that improving the control of the asthma decreases nocturnal symptoms. If it does not, then investigation of potential allergens and a sleep study may be indicated.

Occupational asthma

The diagnosis of occupational asthma depends on establishing sensitization and airway narrowing in response to exposure to a substance found at the workplace or other special environment. The diagnosis may be difficult because the patient may have late rather than immediate responses to the agent and thus symptoms mainly at night. In addition, symptoms can occur in any asthmatic patient in busy situations, which may be present at the workplace. Studies have clearly shown that removal from the agent is needed to stop progression of the disease, but this is often not a practical solution. Every effort must be made, however, to keep the patient away from the sensitizing agent.

Bronchopulmonary aspergillosis

Allergic bronchopulmonary aspergillosis (ABPA) can be regarded as a complication or as a special form of asthma, although it can occur without asthma. It has now been found in many countries, although the prevalence is unknown. Mucoid impaction was also recognized as a complication of asthma, but only in the last 20 years has the relationship between ABPA and mucoid impaction been recognized. The patient usually gives a history of coughing up thick lumps, pellets, or strings of sputum that may have the shape of an airway. The disease is characterized by episodes during which the asthma is more severe and the sputum difficult to produce. There may be chest pain and occasionally fever.

Investigation of the patient is likely to show typical changes on the chest radiograph and sometimes atelectasis or collapse. The changes are often in the upper zones. There is an eosinophilia and elevated levels of circulating IgE. The skin prick tests to *Aspergillus fumigatus* are usually positive, and precipitating antibodies to the fungus are found in the serum. The treatment of ABPA is oral corticosteroids in high doses, which result in a rapid resolution of symptoms, radiologic changes, and the disappearance of sputum plugs. Sometimes long-term treatment with low doses of oral corticosteroids are needed to control the disease. Untreated attacks or severe repeated attacks can lead to bronchiectasis, and death from extensive disease has been described.

OUTCOMES

In the overall management of asthma, most patients are improved because they respond to the drugs. However, the effectiveness of plans such as that described above are not known. Increasingly, emphasis is being placed on quality of life. This can now be measured, and questionnaires that are specific for asthma are being developed. It is unlikely that progress will be made in management until controlled trials of management plans are undertaken in the long term. In the meantime, it is important to watch the mortality figures carefully.

CONCLUSIONS

The management of patients with asthma has precise aims, and there is sufficient knowledge of the causes and natural history of the disease for a logical approach to be used in achieving these aims. There is, however, an absence of data both about the natural history of the disease and about the long-term effects of existing treatments, and it is not known if the currently proposed plans of management are likely to be successful.

Experience suggests that, in the individual patient, the long-term control of the disease is successful only if the patient becomes actively involved in designing and updating his or her own management plan. The plans include careful assessment of the severity and likely causes of the disease and treatment that combines inhaled corticosteroids with avoidance of provoking stimuli. The plan aims to reduce the severity of the disease and, as this is achieved, the doses of drugs are adjusted. In addition, attention must be paid to the factors that aggravate the disease in individual patients.

Emphasis on outcome rests not only on the role of allergens in both causing and exacerbating the disease. Together with the knowledge that persistent asthma is incurable, these considerations are leading to more emphasis being placed on prevention. Prevention of the disease will become the focus of management because its prevalence appears to be increasing and the drugs that are effective in controlling it are affordable by governments or individuals only in affluent countries. In addition, the cost effectiveness of treating asthma is being addressed in many places so that treatment becomes more precise and more logical.

SELECTED REFERENCES

International Consensus Report on the Diagnosis and Treatment of Asthma, National Heart, Lung and Blood Institute, National Institute of Health, Bethesda, MD, 1992. Clin Exp Allergy 1992;22:Suppl 1.

Ortega-Carr D, Bush RK, Busse WW. Evaluation and treatment of the patient with asthma—adult asthma. In: Bierman CW, Pearlman DS, Shapiro GG, Busse WW, eds. Allergy, asthma and immunology from infancy to adulthood. Philadelphia: W.B. Saunders, 1996:498–519.

Mechanisms of Action and Use of β_2-Adrenoceptor Agonists

4

INTRODUCTION

Epinephrine and norepinephrine are adrenal hormones that produce a wide range of biologic actions, many of which are mimicked by the sympathetic nervous system. Classification of the receptors for these compounds into α and β types was crucial to the initial understanding of the actions of these natural catecholamines. Both norepinephrine and epinephrine are potent agonists in many tissues whereas only epinephrine is potent in relaxing airway and vascular smooth muscle. Therefore, existence of subtypes of β-adrenoceptors, termed β_1- and β_2-adrenoceptors, has arisen.

For many years, epinephrine was used as a bronchodilator for the treatment of asthma. The development of isoproterenol, a highly β-selective adrenoceptor agonist, was a significant advance over epinephrine in the treatment of asthma, but both are metabolically unstable. The development of the more stable resorcinol analog metaproterenol was another important advance, but like isoproterenol, metaproterenol produces cardiac side effects. Agonists selective for β_2-adrenoceptors, which produce bronchodilatation without the concomitant tachycardia associated with the earlier compounds, have emerged. The prototype, albuterol, which, despite the subsequent development of terbutaline, fenoterol, clenbuterol, and procaterol (Figure 4-1), is the most widely used of this class of drugs.

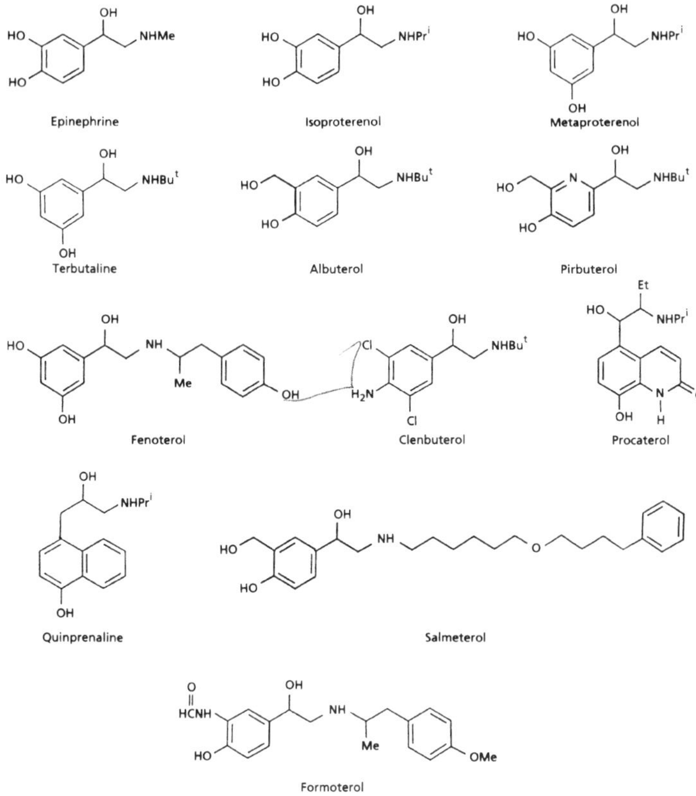

Figure 4-1. Structure of some representative β-adrenoceptor agonists. Reprinted from Busse WW, Holgate ST. Asthma and Rhinitis. Boston: Blackwell Science, 1995.

One shortcoming of the potent, selective β_2-adrenoceptor agonists is their duration of action. In each case, the bronchodilator activity resulting from a single administration of the drug has no more than four hours' duration, and this is clearly inadequate to provide protection from bronchospasm through the night.

Formoterol and salmeterol are two compounds that have a therapeutically significant increased duration of action by the inhaled route of administration. Following inhalation in humans, both exhibit bronchodilator activity for up to 12 hours.

The profile of β-adrenoceptor agonists has been substantially improved since epinephrine, with increased selectivity, first for β-adrenoceptors over α-adrenoceptors, and then for β_2-adrenoceptors over β_1-adrenoceptors. At the same time, enhanced chemical and metabolic stability made this class of compounds far more attractive as drugs, and they have been the mainstay of asthma therapy over the past three decades. Finally, recent improvements in the inherent duration of action of β_2-adrenoceptor agonists have given rise to a new generation of drugs that have the potential for a broader spectrum of bronchodilator and nonbronchodilator properties.

β-ADRENOCEPTOR TRANSDUCTION MECHANISMS

β-Adrenoceptor structure

The cloning of β-adrenoceptors and single amino acid mutation studies have provided a great deal of information as to how β-adrenoceptors function. β-adrenoceptors are members of the family of 7-transmembrane receptors. The human β_2-adrenoceptor is believed to comprise 413 amino acid residues, of approximately 46,480 Da. There are particular amino acid residues that are critical for the binding of β-adrenoceptor agonists to the receptor molecule; three residues are critically important, namely the aspartate (Asp) residue 113 (counted from the extracellular or N-terminus end) and two serine (Ser) residues, 204 and 207. Asp binds to the nitrogen of the β-adrenoceptor agonist molecule, while the two Ser residues interact with the hydroxyl groups on the phenyl ring; although other residues may also be important in agonist recognition, their role has not been fully defined.

Intracellular mediators

β-Adrenoceptors are linked to the enzyme adenylate cyclase, and all of the effects of β-adrenoceptor agonists are mediated by increases in intracellular levels of cyclic $3',5'$-adenosine monophosphate (cAMP). The mechanism by which cAMP induces smooth-muscle-cell relaxation is not fully understood, but cAMP catalyzes the activation of protein kinase A, which in turn results in inhibition of calcium ion (Ca^{2+}), leading to relaxation of the smooth muscle (Figure 4-2).

The coupling of the β-adrenoceptor to adenylate cyclase is affected through a trimeric G protein, which consists of α-, β-, and γ-subunits. Those G proteins linked to β-adrenoceptors are termed G_s, and are stimulatory with respect to adenylate cyclase. β-adrenoceptors exist in two forms, activated and inactivated, and under resting conditions these two forms are in equilibrium, but with the inactivated state being predominant. A receptor is in the

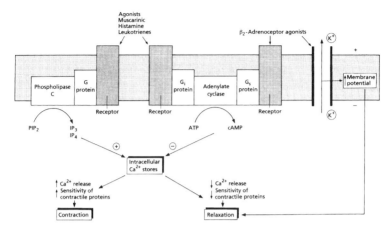

Figure 4-2. Receptor-signal transduction pathways involved in the action of β-adrenoceptor agonists on airway smooth muscle. Reprinted from Busse WW, Holgate ST. Asthma and Rhinitis. Boston: Blackwell Science, 1995.

activated form when it is associated with the α–subunit of the G protein, together with a molecule of guanosine triphosphate (GTP), and it is through this α–subunit that the receptor is coupled to adenylate cyclase. The replacement of the GTP by guanosine diphosphate (GDP) both catalyzes the conversion of ATP to cAMP by the enzyme and dramatically reduces the affinity of the α–subunit for the receptor, resulting in dissociation and causing the receptor to return to its low-energy inactivated form. It is probable that β-agonists achieve their effects not through inducing a conformational change in the receptor, but rather by binding to and temporarily stabilizing receptors in their activated state (i.e., bound to G_s-GTP) and therefore shifting the equilibrium.

Although it has been accepted that β-adrenoceptors are coupled to adenylate cyclase and induce their effects through increases in intracellular cAMP levels, this view has been questioned. This development has followed the observation that some, although not all, effects of β-adrenoceptor agonist stimulation may be inhibited by inhibitors of high-conductance, Ca^{2+}-activated potassium ion (K^+) channels (maxi-K channels). Some data suggest a degree of tissue specificity in transduction processes (see Figure 4-2). There are important questions still to be answered with regard to the mechanisms involved in the transduction of β-adrenoceptor-mediated effects.

Desensitization

Associated with β–adrenoceptor activation is the autoregulatory process of receptor desensitization. This process acts as a safety device to prevent overstimulation of receptors in the face of excessive β–agonist exposure. Desensitization occurs in response to the association of receptor with agonist molecule. The mechanisms by which desensitization can occur appear to consist of three main processes: 1) uncoupling of the receptors from adenylate cyclase, 2) internalization of uncoupled receptors, and 3) phosphorylation of internalized receptors. The extent of desensitization depends on the degree and duration of the β–adrenoceptor/β–agonist response. Thus, simple uncoupling is a transient process and may be reversed within minutes of removal of the agonist. Internalization takes longer to reverse, but full reversal normally occurs within hours. However, phosphorylation may or may not be reversible and is dependent on either dephosphorylation or de nove synthesis of new β–adrenoceptors. The process of desensitization to β–agonists differs markedly from tissue to tissue (e.g., human lymphocytes desensitize very rapidly on exposure to β–agonists whereas human bronchial smooth muscle is resistant). This difference is manifested in the well-documented decline in the side effects associated with β–adrenoceptor agonist therapy (e.g., tachycardia and physiologic tremor) in asthmatic patients, but bronchodilatation is maintained despite regular treatment for prolonged periods.

PHARMACOLOGIC PROFILE OF β_2-AGONISTS

Long-acting β_2-adrenoceptor agonists

Considerable work has been done to develop long-acting β_2-agonists that would be suitable for treatment two times daily. Salmeterol was developed so that it would persist at its binding site(s) and be long acting by continuously interacting with the active site of the β–adrenoceptor. In contrast, formoterol was developed by investigating β–agonist analogs with increased affinity for the β–adrenoceptor itself.

Albuterol and terbutaline are highly hydrophilic in nature, whereas salmeterol is much more lipophilic. The lipophilicity of the β–agonist determines the degree of partitioning into the cell membrane and subsequent diffusion kinetics in interacting with the β–adrenoceptor. In the case of albuterol, the drug accesses the active site of the β–adrenoceptor directly (Figure 4-3) and there is a rapid onset of effect, but, since it is readily removed by diffusion

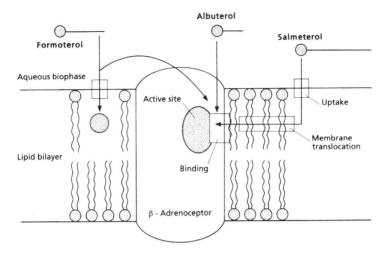

Figure 4-3. Model for the interaction of albuterol, formoterol, and salmeterol with the β-adrenoceptor. Reprinted from Busse WW, Holgate ST. Asthma and Rhinitis. Boston: Blackwell Science, 1995.

into the aqueous phase, the duration of action is short. With lipophilic drugs (e.g., salmeterol), the molecule approaches the active site of the β-adrenoceptor through the outer phospholipid monolayer of the membrane (see Figure 4-3). Although both salmeterol and formoterol have been subjected to considerable experimental scrutiny, there is still no consensus regarding how they achieve their prolonged durations of action. Owing to its relatively lipophilic nature, formoterol partitions extensively into the cell membrane, which effectively acts as a reservoir for the drug (see Figure 4-3).

β_2-Adrenoceptor selectivity

β_1-Adrenoceptors are mainly located in the heart, whereas β_2-adrenoceptors are more widespread, found in airways and vascular smooth muscle, leukocytes, endothelial cells, epithelial cells, and mast cells. The aim of bronchodilator therapy is to produce an optimal airway response with minimal systemic adverse effects. The latter may be divided into those that are β_2-adrenoceptor mediated and include skeletal muscle tremor, hypokalemia, and electrocardiographic changes, as well as those such as heart rate that appear to be the result of direct stimulation of both β_1- and β_2-adrenoceptors.

61

Neither of the naturally occurring catecholamines, epinephrine and norepinephrine, is selective for β-adrenoceptors, since these compounds also exhibit α-adrenoceptor agonist activity. Substantial modifications to the N-substituent of the natural catecholamines have resulted in a range of potent β-adrenoceptor selective agonists, some of which also demonstrate a degree of β_2-adrenoceptor selectivity.

A catechol ring is not essential for β_2-adrenoceptor agonist activity. This was initially demonstrated with modifications to produce resorcinols, such as metaproterenol, terbutaline, and fenoterol, and saligenins, such as albuterol and salmeterol (see Figure 4-1). More extensive modifications to the phenyl ring involved replacing the *meta* hydroxyl (OH) group with alternative structures, such as methane sulfonamide (e.g., soterenol), urea (e.g., carbuterol), and formylamide (e.g., formoterol). With the exception of the resorcinols, such modifications *per se* seemed to confer a degree of β_2-adrenoceptor selectivity on the molecules. Even a phenyl ring is not an essential requirement for a β_2-adrenoceptor agonist; for example, in pirbuterol, the ring structure is a pyridine, and in others the phenyl ring has been replaced with a bicyclic structure such as carbostyryl (procaterol).

β_2-Adrenoceptor agonists vary widely in potency, from metaproterenol, albuterol, and terbutaline, which are at least tenfold weaker than isproterenol, to formoterol and procaterol, which are approximately 20-fold more potent than isoproterenol. Not only do the absolute potencies of the compounds at β_2-adrenoceptors vary considerably, but their degrees of selectivity for β_2-adrenoceptors with respect to β_1-adrenoceptors also differ markedly. For example, at cardiac β_1-adrenoceptors all β_2-agonists are less potent than isoproterenol, but this ranges from 20-fold for fenoterol to more than 10,000-fold for salmeterol. Salmeterol is the most selective β_2-adrenoceptor agonist identified to date (Table 4-1).

Affinity and efficacy

Most β-adrenoceptor agonists have a rather low affinity for their receptors. Few β_2-agonists have been shown to have a much higher affinity than isoproterenol, but among these are procaterol, formoterol, and salmeterol. Albuterol, in contrast, has a relatively low affinity for β_2-adrenoceptors.

β-Adrenoceptor potency is a function not only of receptor affinity but also of receptor efficacy. The difference between a β-

Table 4-1. Comparative β-Adrenoceptor Selectivity of a Range of β-Agonists

β-Agonist	Relative potency			Selectivity ratio*	
	β_1-Adrenoceptors (atria: inotropic activity)	β_2-Adrenoceptors (bronchus: relaxant activity)	β_3-Adrenoceptors (adipocytes: lipolytic activity)	$\beta_2:\beta_1$	$\beta_2:\beta_3$
Isoproterenol	1.0	1.0	1.0	1.0	1.0
Albuterol	0.0004	0.55	0.002	1375	275
Fenoterol	0.005	0.6	0.02	120	30
Formoterol	0.05	20.0	0.065	400	305
Salmeterol	0.0001	8.5	0.009	85,000	945

*Derived by dividing the relative potency at β_2-adrenoceptors by the corresponding potency at β_1- or β_3-adrenoceptors.

Table 4-2. Relative Potency, Time of Onset, and Duration of Action of β₂-Adrenoceptor Agonists in Relaxing Inherent Tone in the Human Superfused Bronchus Preparation in Vitro

	Relative potency	Onset time (min)	Duration of action (min)
Isoproterenol	1.0	1.5	2.2
Albuterol	0.1	3.3	6.9
Formoterol	7.8	2.1	6.6
Salmeterol	11.6	35.6	>240

agonist and a β-antagonist is not absolute, but rather one of degree; thus, both have affinity for the receptor, but different efficacies. A "full agonist" has a high efficacy, while a "pure antagonist" has low efficacy. The majority of β_2-adrenoceptor agonists have an intermediate efficacy. If receptor density is too low or coupling is inadequate, the β-agonist may behave in a "partial" manner (i.e., it will be incapable of achieving the same maximum effect as an agonist of higher efficacy). Examples of compounds with high efficacy (approximately equivalent to isoproterenol) are procaterol and formoterol, whereas most saligenins and resorcinols—albuterol, salmeterol, and terbutaline, for example—tend to be of moderate efficacy (65 to 85% of that of isoproterenol). The efficacy of β_2-agonists at extrapulmonary β-adrenoceptors may be of clinical importance. For example, fenoterol and formoterol have the same efficacy as isoproterenol at cardiac β_1 adrenoceptors, but albuterol is a partial agonist and salmeterol has very low efficacy.

Onset and duration of action

There are differences in the rate of onset and duration of action of β_2-agonists (Table 4-2). In human bronchial smooth muscle in vitro, the onset of action of isoproterenol, albuterol, terbutaline, and fenoterol is rapid (<4 min), that of formoterol is somewhat delayed (>6 min), and responses to salmeterol are slow to reach equilibrium under these conditions (>30 min). These differences are not so apparent clinically, however, where, for example, the time to 15% increase in the forced expiratory volume in one second (FEV_1) following a 50-μg dose of salmeterol is only a few minutes slower than that with a standard 200-μg dose of albuterol. In contrast, there are marked differences in the duration of action of β_2-agonists. While isoproterenol has a short duration of action, and equipotent concentrations of albuterol and formoterol are similar, the relaxant effects of salmeterol on airway smooth muscle are long lasting. The duration of action of β_2-agonists in the human bronchus is in this order: salmeterol $\gg$ formoterol $\geq$ albuterol $\geq$ terbutaline $>$ fenoterol.

BRONCHODILATOR ACTIVITY

Episodic bronchoconstriction and airway hyperreactivity are two of the cardinal features of asthma. Bronchoconstriction can arise by a number of mechanisms, including direct activation of bronchial smooth muscle by locally generated mediators, stimulation of neurogenic pathways in the airways, and extravasation of plasma proteins into lung tissue, leading to edema formation and narrowing of the airway lumen.

To date, β_2-agonists have been the most successful approach to controlling bronchospasm in asthma. Albuterol and other selective β_2-adrenoceptor agonists have proven to be highly efficacious and well tolerated over many years of clinical use. The major drawback with the first-generation drugs is their duration of action of four to six hours, which limits their usefulness in controlling the symptoms of nocturnal asthma and in providing convenient maintenance therapy for the patient. This problem has been overcome with the new generation of long-acting β_2-agonists represented by salmeterol and formoterol.

Airway smooth muscle

In isolated airway preparations, all β-agonists relax the tissue either when tone is induced with a spasmogen—prostaglandin (PGF_{2a}), histamine, carbachol—or by electrical field stimulation. Contractions may result from direct stimulation of the muscle or be of cholinergic, sympathetic, or nonadrenergic-noncholinergic origin, in which case the β-agonist may exert its relaxant effects at the pre- and/or postjunctional level. Alternatively, where antigen-induced contractions are due to the release of spasmogenic mediators, the relaxant activity of a β-agonist may then result from either functional antagonism or inhibition of mediator release. The maximal degree of relaxation induced by salmeterol is consistently less than that of isoproterenol and albuterol, indicating the partial agonist nature of the response. Albuterol, fenoterol, and formoterol all have a short duration of action, but this can be prolonged by increasing the concentration of the β-agonist applied to the tissue. The profile of salmeterol is very different, with a duration of effect in excess of seven hours, and this is independent of the concentration used. These differences among β-agonists are also apparent in human airways (see Table 4-2).

Clinical experience with long-acting β_2-agonists

The long-acting β_2-adrenoceptor agonists were developed specifically for inhaled use as two times daily maintenance therapy in the treatment of reversible airway obstruction. The early clinical studies have shown that salmeterol and formoterol produce dose-dependent bronchodilatation in asthmatic patients with longer durations of action than albuterol; furthermore, salmeterol protected against methacholine challenge and exercise-induced asthma for at least 12 hours.

Both salmeterol and formoterol have also been evaluated for their efficacy in clinical asthma and produce significant increases in both morning and evening peak flow. They also reduce both the diurnal variation in lung function and nocturnal symptoms. These effects were sustained for three months of treatment, with no evidence of loss of response.

β_2-Agonists are therefore potent and effective as bronchodilator drugs against a wide range of bronchoconstrictor stimuli. The major drawback of the first-generation drugs, such as albuterol, was duration of action; this has been overcome with the second-generation long-acting β-agonists, salmeterol and formoterol. In practice, the dose range of even highly selective β_2-agonists is often limited by extrapulmonary side effects mediated by systemic β_2-adrenoceptors. The therapeutic index of β_2-agonists can be improved by administration via the inhaled, as opposed to the oral, route.

NONBRONCHODILATOR PROPERTIES

The pharmacologic activity of β_2-agonists is not restricted to airway smooth muscle, and these agents also exhibit a range of nonbronchodilator properties. For example, there is experimental evidence that β-agonists can inhibit acute inflammatory responses in the lung. Clinical experience, however, has not shown currently available β_2-agonists to have significant anti-inflammatory activity in the lung. Indeed, whereas it is generally recognized that drugs such as albuterol and terbutaline are effective against immediate bronchospasm resulting from allergen challenge, they have little, if any, effect on the late response or the accompanying increase in bronchial hyperreactivity.

Mast cells and inflammatory mediator release

Functional β-adrenoceptors have been detected in lung mast cells, and β_2-agonists inhibit release of inflammatory mediators (histamine, leukotrienes, prostaglandins) from these cells. The rank order of potency in inhibiting mast cell mediator release is formoterol $>$ salmeterol $\geq$ isoproterenol $>$ albuterol, but all of the drugs are capable of producing complete inhibition of mediator release. Importantly, the concentration range for this effect is the same as that which relaxes human airway smooth muscle. However, in contrast to short-acting β_2-agonists, which are active for only up to four hours, salmeterol has a sustained effect, suppressing histamine, leukotriene C_4 (LTC_4), and D_4 and prostaglandin D_2 release for >20 hours, while the duration of action of formoterol (eight hours) is intermediate between that of salmeterol and albuterol.

An effect of β_2-agonists on mast-cell-derived mediator release has also been demonstrated in vivo following antigen challenge of sensitized subjects. However, in these studies, albuterol was shown to inhibit only the acute rise in circulating histamine and neutrophil chemotactic factor or urinary LTE_4 and, in the context of potential anti-inflammatory activity of β_2-agonists in the lung, a long duration of mediator inhibition may be important.

Endothelial cells: vascular permeability

Inflammatory mediators interact with specific receptors on vascular endothelial cells, particularly in postcapillary venules, to induce contraction and the opening of the tight junctions between adjacent cells leading to tissue edema. Increased intracellular cAMP may maintain the integrity of the vascular endothelium, thereby limiting plasma protein extravasation.

The duration of action for the effect of β_2-agonists on vascular permeability in the lung is in the rank order salmeterol > formoterol > albuterol. The limiting step in resolving tissue edema is not only the rate of extravasation, but the rate of clearance of the interstitial protein. The duration of action of β_2-agonists in inhibiting vascular permeability may therefore be of critical importance in determining their activity against this aspect of acute inflammation. A transient reduction in plasma protein extravasation, such as would result from the action of a short-acting β-agonist, would not have a substantial antiedema effect. In contrast, a long-acting β_2-agonist that inhibits vascular permeability changes in the lung for up to eight hours after a single inhaled dose may be capable of limiting protein and water leakage from the vasculature for a sufficient period to allow tissue clearance mechanisms to be effective.

Inflammatory cells

Although this is not proven, β_2-agonists may inhibit the accumulation of granulocytes at sites of acute inflammation. β_2-Agonists may also inhibit inflammatory cell recruitment, by limiting the release of chemotactic mediators, but this is unlikely to be the only mechanism of action. Alternatively, an effect on the vascular endothelium, in addition to attenuating plasma protein extravasation, may be operative. β_2-Agonists such as albuterol and salmeterol increase the intracellular cAMP concentration in endothelial cells in culture, thereby maintaining the integrity of the endothelium and inhibiting the recruitment of inflammatory cells.

Bronchial epithelium

The bronchial epithelium also contains functional β-adrenoceptors, and β_2-agonists may, therefore, also be effective in modulating some of the consequences of acute inflammation at the level of the epithelium. Cilia play a major role in preserving the functional integrity of the airways, particularly as part of the clearance mechanisms for excessive airway secretions that occur in response to inflammatory stimuli. Efficient clearance of mucus is dependent on coordinated patterns of ciliary activity and the total numbers of cilia involved. Both abnormal mucus production and defects in mucociliary clearance occur in asthma. Neurohormones and neurotransmitters influence mucociliary clearance by modifying the cilial beat frequency through changes in epithelial cell calcium and cAMP.

Albuterol and salmeterol increase cilial beat frequency in human bronchial epithelial cells in culture, with salmeterol being more potent than albuterol. The effects of albuterol are modest and transient in nature, whereas salmeterol produced an increment in cilial beat frequency in bronchial epithelium, and its effect was sustained for 15 to 20 hours.

Clinical studies

Long-acting β_2-agonists inhibit a number of the processes involved in acute inflammation. They could potentially represent a new class of anti-inflammatory drugs, acting directly as functional antagonists to inhibit inflammatory mediator release, plasma protein extravasation, and inflammatory cell accumulation, and with the possibility of maintaining their effects on a 24-hour basis by dosing two times daily. They should not be seen as replacements for steroids, but rather as complementary to existing anti-inflammatory therapy since there is no evidence they control the chronic airway inflammation seen in asthma.

β_2-Agonists therefore have pharmacologic effects against both the process and the consequences of acute inflammation in the lung. These effects are seen with the new long-acting drugs or with high or repeated doses of short-acting compounds and arise from prolonged activation of β-adrenoceptors in a range of target cells. Under these conditions, the profile of anti-inflammatory activity of the β_2-agonists is at least comparable with that of other prophylactic drugs such as disodium cromoglycate, ketotifen, and theophylline. Further clinical work is clearly necessary before the clinical significance of the nonbronchodilator effects of the long-acting β_2-agonists in bronchial asthma can be evaluated.

CLINICAL USE OF β_2-ADRENORECEPTOR AGONISTS

β-Adrenoreceptor agonists are currently the most potent and effective bronchodilators available. Inhaled β-agonists are the treatment of choice for acute smooth muscle–mediated bronchoconstriction in asthma.

Emergency department use

At the present time, nebulized therapy is used for most instances where emergency treatment for acute exacerbations of asthma is required. Albuterol and metaproterenol are the most frequently used agents, with albuterol often chosen for its slightly longer duration of action and more β₂-selectivity. Typically, for adults 2.5 mg of albuterol (0.5 ml of a 0.5% solution in 2.5 ml of normal saline) or for children 0.1 to 0.15 mg/kg/dose is given every 20 minutes for 60 minutes (three doses) and then hourly during the first several hours of therapy. For severely obstructed patients, 0.5 mg/kg/hr can be given by continuous nebulization.

Some studies suggest that giving two to eight puffs of an intermediate-acting β-agonist by metered-dose inhaler with a spacer device is as effective as a nebulized treatment. Many clinicians, however, use nebulizer therapy since less instruction and coordination is required (Table 4-3 and Table 4-4).

Epinephrine 0.3 mg subcutaneously (0.01 mg/kg/dose up to 0.3 to 0.5 mg for children) or subcutaneous terbutaline (0.25 mg) have been used if nebulizer therapy is not available or ineffective (see Table 4-3 and Table 4-4). Caution is indicated for adults older than 40 years or in patients with known cardiac disease.

Intravenous use of β-agonists is rarely indicated but may be considered on an individual basis in patients under 40 years of age who have not responded to nebulized therapy and in whom respiratory arrest is imminent. Isoproterenol has been associated with adverse cardiac events and therefore is to be avoided.

Table 4-3. Doses* of Drugs in Acute Exacerbations of Asthma in Adults

Inhaled β-agonist nebulizer solutions (see text)
- Albuterol 2.5 mg (0.5 cc of a 0.5% solution, diluted with 2–3 cc of normal saline)

or

- Metaproterenol 15 mg (0.3 cc of a 5% solution, diluted with 2–3 cc of normal saline)

Subcutaneous β-agonists (see text)
- Epinephrine 0.3 mg s.q.

or

- Terbutaline 0.25 mg s.q.

---

*Administered every 20 minutes for 60 minutes (three doses).
Adapted from National Heart, Lung, and Blood Institute Guidelines, 1991.

Table 4-4. Doses of Drugs in Acute Exacerbations of Asthma in Children

Drug	Available from	Dose	Comment
Inhaled β₂-agonist			
Albuterol			
Metered-dose inhaler	90 µg/puff	2 inhalations every 5 min for total of 12 puffs, with monitoring of PEFR or FEV₁ to document response	If not improved, switch to nebulizer. If improved, decrease to 4 puffs every hour.
Nebulizer solution	0.5% (5 mg/ml)	0.1–0.15 mg/kg/dose up to 5 mg every 20 min for 1–2 hrs (minimum dose 1.25 mg/dose); 0.5 mg/kg/hr by continuous nebulization (maximum 15 mg/hour)	If improved, decrease to every 1–2 hours. If not improved, use by continuous inhalation.
Metaproterenol			
Metered-dose inhaler	650 µg/puff	2 inhalations	Frequent high-dose administration has not been evaluated. Metaproterenol is not interchangeable with β₂-agonists albuterol and terbutaline.
Nebulizer solution	5% (50 mg/ml)	0.1–0.3 cc (5–15 mg). Do not exceed 15 mg	
	0.6% unit dose vial of 2.5 ml (15 mg)	As above, 5–15 mg. Do not exceed 15 mg	

Terbutaline			
Metered-dose inhaler	200 μg/puff	2 inhalations every 5 min for a total of 12 puffs	
Injectable solution used in nebulizer	0.1% (1 mg/1 ml) solution in 0.9% NaCl solution for injection. Not FDA approved for inhalation.		Not recommended since not available as nebulizer solution. Offers no advantage over albuterol, which is available as nebulizer solution.
Systemic β-agonist			
Epinephrine HCl	1:1000 (1 mg/ml)	0.01 mg/kg up to 0.3 mg subcutaneously every 20 minutes for 3 doses	Inhaled β₂-agonist preferred.
Terbutaline	(0.1%) 1 mg/ml solution for injection in 0.9% NaCl	Subcutaneous 0.01 mg/kg up to 0.3 mg every 2–6 hours as needed. Intravenous 10 μg/kg over 10 minutes loading dose. Maintenance: 0.4 μg/kg/min. Increase as necessary by 0.2 μg/kg/min and expect to use 3–6 μg/kg/min.	Inhaled β₂-agonist preferred.

Adapted from National Heart, Lung, and Blood Institute Guidelines, 1991.

Treatment of the hospitalized asthmatic

Once a patient with status asthmaticus is hospitalized, continued therapy with inhaled β-agonists is usually indicated. Nebulized β-agonists (e.g., nebulized albuterol 2.5 mg for adults) can be given every one to two hours and increased in frequency to every 30 minutes in patients with severe disease (Figure 4-4). Albuterol 0.15 mg/kg/hr is given every one to two hours for children in severe distress; continuous albuterol nebulization (0.5 mg/kg/hr; maximum 15 mg/hr) may be considered as well as intravenous terbutaline (10 μg/kg loading dose, then 0.4 mg/kg/min up to 3–6 μg/kg/min) (Figure 4-5).

Outpatient management of chronic asthma

Fortunately, most patients with asthma do not require emergency treatment or hospitalization. For the majority of patients metered-dose immediate-acting β-agonist is a foundation of therapy.

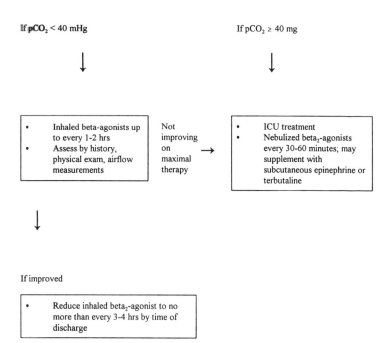

Figure 4-4.   Use of β-Agonists in Acute Exacerbations of Asthma in Adults—Hospital Management.

If PEFR > 30% baseline and/or pCO$_2$ < 40 mHg,

O$_2$ sat. $\geq$ 90%

If PEFR < 30% baseline, and/or

pCO$_2$ $\geq$ 40 mmHg, O$_2$ Sat. < 90%

↓ ↓

	Not		
• Monitored unit • Nebulized albuterol 0.15 mg/kg/dose every 1-2 hrs	improved on maximal therapy →	• ICU • Continuous nebulized albuterol 0.5 mg/kg/hr - max 15 mg/hr	

↓ ↓

If improved

If not improving

↓ ↓

• Decrease frequency of nebulized albuterol	Consider IV terbutaline

Figure 4-5. Use of β-Agonists in Acute Exacerbations of Asthma in Children—Hospital Management.

Exercise-induced asthma

Exercise is a potent stimulus to bronchoconstriction in most asthmatics. Treatment is instituted with two puffs of an intermediate-acting β$_2$-agonist prior to exercise (Figure 4-6). If the patient experiences symptoms, two puffs are administered for relief. At the next exercise period, the dose of the β-agonist may be increased to four puffs in order to prevent bronchoconstriction. The long-acting β-agonist salmeterol has been shown to inhibit exercise-induced asthma symptoms for up to 12 hours. Its use should be limited to two puffs prior to exercise, and it must be given at least one hour before the activity to reach maximum effect. Since its onset of action is delayed, it is not useful if breakthrough symptoms

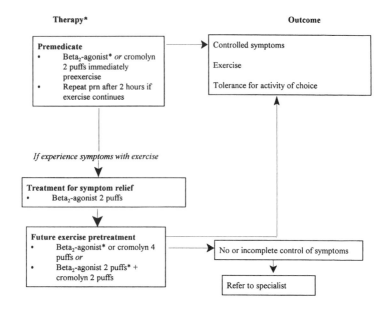

*or salmeterol 2 puffs 1 hr before exercise

Figure 4-6. Use of β-Agonists in Exercise-induced Asthma.

occur. Therefore, intermediate-acting β-agonists are more useful for both prophylaxis and treatment of exercise-induced asthma symptoms.

Finally, in some well-conditioned athletes who participate in long-duration activities (e.g., marathon runners, cross-country ski racers), nebulized therapy with a β-agonist and/or cromolyn or nedocrimil may be necessary for effective control.

Chronic asthma

For patients with mild asthma, the use of a metered-dose inhaled β-agonist for symptoms up to twice a week is considered adequate therapy (Table 4-5 and Table 4-6). For patients with more frequent symptoms, the use of an immediate-acting β-agonist up to three to four times a day combined with anti-inflammatory therapy is appropriate. However, if symptom control requires the use of the intermediate-acting β-agonist so often and/or nocturnal symptoms occur, the use of a long-acting β-agonist such as salmeterol (two puffs twice a day) should be considered. Oral β-agonists may also be considered, but their use has largely been supplanted by the long-acting inhaled β-agonists.

Table 4-5. β_2-Agonists in the Management of Adult Asthma

Chronic mild asthma	Chronic moderate asthma	Chronic severe asthma
Asymptomatic		
Pretreat prn 1–2 puffs immediate acting β_2-agonist for exercise, allergen, or other stimuli	Inhaled, immediate-acting β_2-agonist prn to TID/QID and anti-inflammatory agent	Inhaled, immediate-acting β_2-agonist and anti-inflammatory agent
	↓	↓
Symptomatic		
Inhaled, intermediate-acting β_2-agonist (2 puffs repeated every 3–4 hrs prn for duration of episode)	If sx persist, consider salmeterol 2 puffs BID or oral β_2-agonist	If sx persist, salmeterol 2 puffs BID, episodic extra β_2-agonist (2–4 puffs MDI or nebulized) for exacerbation

Adapted from National Heart, Lung, and Blood Institute Guidelines, 1991.

Table 4-6. Use of β-Agonists in Childhood Asthma

Chronic mild asthma	Chronic moderate asthma	Chronic severe asthma
Asymptomatic	Inhaled, immediate-acting β_2-agonist prn to TID/QID	Inhaled, intermediate-acting β_2-agonist prn to TID/QID
Pretreat prn 1–2 puffs immediate-acting β_2-agonist for exercise, allergen, or other stimuli	and cromolyn or → nedocromil or → Inhaled β_2-agonist prn and salmeterol 2 puffs BID	If <5 yrs nebulized If >5 yrs inhaled 2 puffs or 1 inhaled dry powder capsule QID or every 4 hrs and anti-inflammatory agent
Symptomatic		
If <5 yrs nebulized or oral	If sx persist, inhaled corticosteroids	If sx persist, 2 puffs salmeterol BID or oral β_2-agonist
If >5 yrs inhaled 2 puffs or 1 inhaled dry powder capsule intermediate-acting β_2-agonist every 4–6 hrs prn for duration of the episode		Episodic either β_2-agonist (2–4 puffs MDI or nebulized) or intermediate acting β_2-agonist for exacerbations

Adapted from National Heart, Lung, and Blood Institute Guidelines, 1991.

Table 4-7. Dosages of β_2-Agonists for Therapy in Childhood Asthma

Inhaled

Examples: Albuterol, metaproterenol, bitolterol, terbutaline, pirbuteral

Metered-dose inhaler	2 puffs q 4–6 hours
Dry powder inhaler	1 capsule q 4–6 hours
Nebulizer solution★	Albuterol 5 mg/ml; 0.1–0.15 mg/ kg in 2 cc of saline q 4–6 hours, maximum 5.0 mg
	Metaproterenol 50 mg/ml; 0.25–0.50 mg/kg in 2 cc of saline q 4–6 hours, maximum 15.0 mg

Oral

Liquids	Albuterol	0.1–0.15 mg/kg q 4–6 hours
	Metaproterenol	0.3–0.5 mg/kg q 4–6 hours
Tablets	Albuterol	2 or 4 mg tablet, q 4–6 hours
		4 mg sustained-release tablet q 12 hours
	Metaproterenol	10 or 20 mg tablet q 4–6 hours
	Terbutaline	2.5 or 5.0 mg tablet q 4–6 hours

★ Premixed solutions are available—follow dosages as above.
Adapted from National Heart, Lung, and Blood Institute Guidelines, 1991.

In children who are unable to coordinate the use of a metered-dose inhaler, nebulizer therapy or oral forms of β-agonists may be used (Table 4-7; see also Table 4-6).

Currently, there is controversy as to whether or not regular daily use of β-agonists is harmful. Clearly, the use of more than one canister of an intermediate-acting β-agonist per month by a patient is a marker for severe disease. Excessive or increased use of a β-agonist warrants consideration of additional (anti-inflammatory) therapy. Patients should reduce nonessential use of intermediate-acting β-agonists to premedication for prophylaxis of exercise-induced asthma and limit their use to "rescue" for breakthrough symptoms.

CONCLUSIONS

Although, as a class, β-adrenoceptor agonists share a number of pharmacologic properties, there are marked differences in receptor affinity, efficacy, selectivity, and duration of action among individual compounds. The optimal pharmacologic profile is represented by a drug that is lipophilic, in order to increase occupancy at the β-adrenoceptor and to promote retention in the lung, leading to decreased systemic absorption and therefore fewer extrapulmonary side effects. The drug should be both potent and highly β_2-adrenoceptor selective and ideally have an intrinsically long duration of action at β-adrenoceptors without causing tachyphylaxis.

The objective of developing a drug with long-lasting bronchodilator activity for the treatment of reversible airways obstruction has been achieved in the new generation of β-agonists, represented by salmeterol and formoterol. Both are potent and highly selective β_2-agonists but appear to have different mechanisms of action. Clinical studies have confirmed that they are well tolerated and highly efficacious, providing bronchodilation in asthmatic patients for at least 12 hours. The pharmacologic profile of the two drugs results from their ability to produce prolonged activation of β_2-adrenoceptors in a range of target cells, including not only airway smooth muscle, but also mast cells, vascular endothelial cells, and bronchial epithelial cells. Their profile of activity extends to include nonbronchodilator properties, such as suppression of inflammatory mediator release, inhibition of vascular permeability, and attenuation of inflammatory cell recruitment, processes involved in acute inflammation in the lung. Additional studies are now required to establish whether this nonbronchodilator activity of the long-acting β_2-adrenoceptor agonists has clinical relevance in bronchial asthma, either in terms of monotherapy or as an adjunct to inhaled corticosteroids.

SELECTED REFERENCES

Barnes PJ. Beta-adrenergic receptors and their regulation. Am J Respir Crit Care Med 1995;152:838–860.

Boulet L-P. Long versus short-acting β_2-agonists. Implications for drug therapy. Drugs 1994;207:207–222.

Gern JE, Lemanske RF Jr. β-adrenergic agonist therapy. Immunol Allergy Clin No Amer 1993;13:839–860.

McFadden ER Jr. Prospectives in β_2-agonist therapy. vox clamantis in deserto vel lux in tenebris? J Allergy Clin Immunol 1995;95:641–651.

National Heart, Lung and Blood Institute. International consensus report on diagnosis and management of asthma. Eur Respir J 1992;5:601–641.

Nelson H. β-adrenergic bronchodilators. N Engl J Med 1995;333:499–506.

Mechanisms of Action and Clinical Use of Glucocorticoids in Asthma

5

I. MECHANISMS OF ACTION OF GLUCOCORTICOIDS

INTRODUCTION

Glucocorticoids, first reported to be useful in the treatment of asthma over 40 years ago, have numerous biochemical and physiological actions that may contribute to their efficacy. This chapter will discuss the proposed mechanisms of action for glucocorticoids, specifically their effects on the various inflammatory cells, cell trafficking and chemotaxis, mediator synthesis and release, vascular permeability, β-adrenergic receptor activity, and bronchial hyperreactivity. The chemistry and pharmacokinetics of the various glucocorticoids administered systemically and topically in the treatment of asthma and rhinitis will also be discussed.

CHEMISTRY AND STRUCTURE ACTIVITY RELATIONSHIPS

First isolated over 60 years ago, cortisone was found to have efficacy in the treatment of asthma (Figure 5-1). Subsequent structural modifications have successfully separated the mineralocorticoid from the metabolic and anti-inflammatory effects; however, it has not been possible to isolate the desired anti-inflammatory properties from undesirable metabolic effects. All anti-inflammatory steroids have a 2 carbon chain at the 17 position and methyl groups

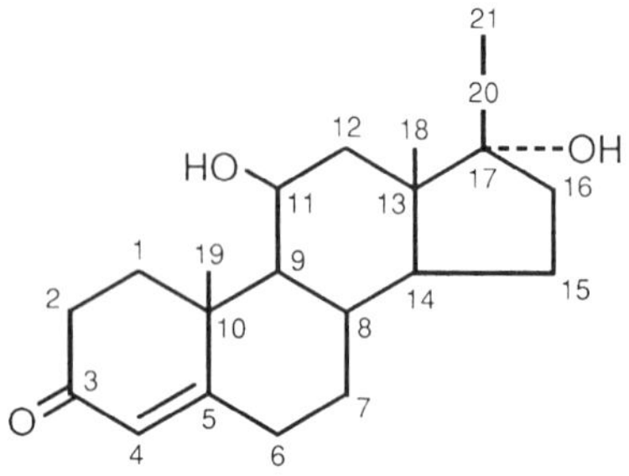

Figure 5-1. The Basic Glucocorticoid Structure with Carbon Atoms Numbered.

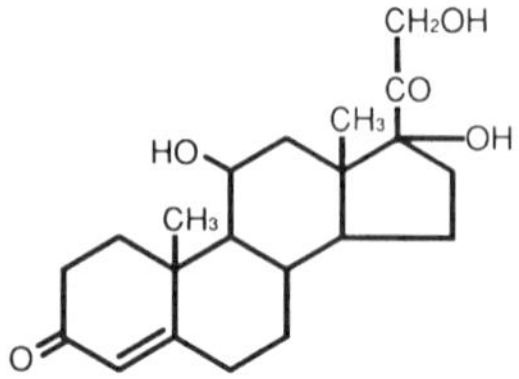

hydrocortisone

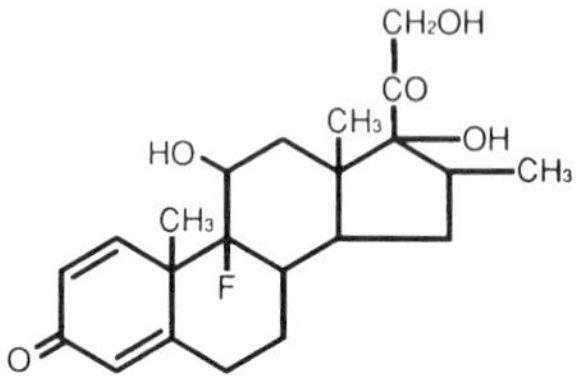

dexamethasone

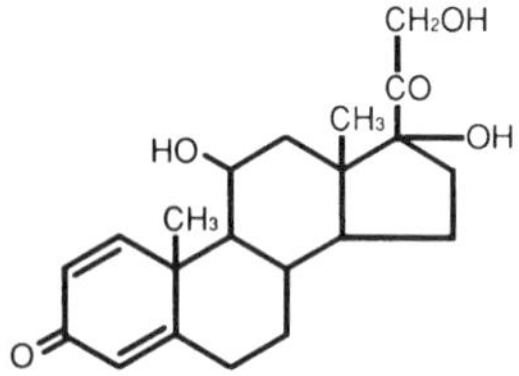

prednisolone

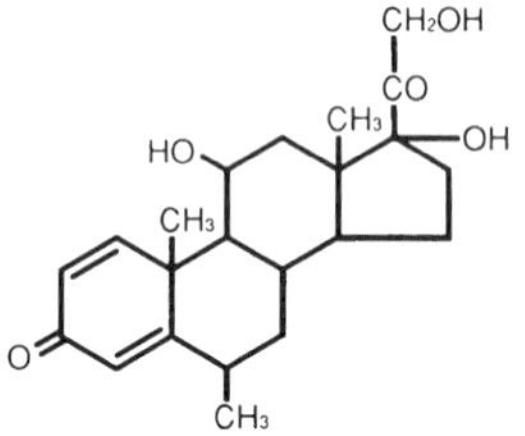

methylprednisolone

Figure 5-2. Chemical Structure of Commonly Used Systemically Administered Glucocorticoids.

at carbons 18 and 19 (Figure 5-2). Other essential features necessary for activity consist of a ketone at carbons 3 and 20, a double bond between carbons 4 and 5, and a hydroxyl group at carbon 11. Modifications to the basic steroid structure have increased anti-inflammatory properties while decreasing mineralocorticoid effects. Addition of a double bond at the 1,2 position, resulting in prednisolone, and the addition of a methyl group at the number 6 carbon, resulting in methylprednisolone, are examples. Fluorination of the number 9 carbon, as with dexamethasone, is associated with increasing systemic glucocorticoid potency by a factor of 25 when compared to hydrocortisone, without a major increase in topical potency (Table 5-1).

Topical activity

Glucocorticoids with a high degree of topical activity suitable for pulmonary or nasal application have been synthesized primarily by replacement of hydroxyl groups at carbons 16 and 17 with acetal groups, as with triamcinolone acetonide and flunisolide (Figure 5-3). Beclomethasone dipropionate differs slightly, with a propionate ester substituted at carbons 17 and 21 and a chlorine at carbon 9 (see Figure 5-3). Glucocorticoids being introduced into clinical trials for inhalation or intranasal administration include mometasone furoate (Schering-Plough), which contains a 16 methyl and a furan ring ester at carbon 17 in addition to a carbon 9 chlorine. Fluticasone propionate (Glaxo), which has a 17 carbon propionate substitution and a 21 carbon thiofluoromethyl ester, is currently available as a nasal spray for rhinitis and as a metered-dose inhaler in 3-dose formulations for asthma therapy. Fluticasone also has two fluorine substitutions at carbons 6 and 9. One of the newest topical glucocorticoids, tipredane (Fisons), is available in Europe. This unique compound has two alkylthio substitutes at carbon 17 in place of the hydroxyl and 2 carbon side chain of cortisol. Similar to other glucocorticoids used in the treatment of asthma and rhinitis, tipredane has a halogen substitution with a fluorine at carbon 9. Budesonide is the only topically active antiasthma glucocorticoid lacking the carbon 9 halogenation; its only difference from

Table 5-1. Relative Potencies of Commonly Used Systemic Glucocorticoids

Glucocorticoid	Relative anti-inflammatory potency	Equivalent dose (mg)
Hydrocortisone	1	20
Dexamethasone	30	0.75
Methylprednisolone	5	4
Prednisolone	4	5

Source Ellul-Micallef R. Pharmacokinetics and pharmacodynamics of glucocorticosteroids. In: Jenne JW, Murphy S, eds. Drug therapy for asthma. Research and clinical practice. New York: Marcel Dekker, 1987:463–516.

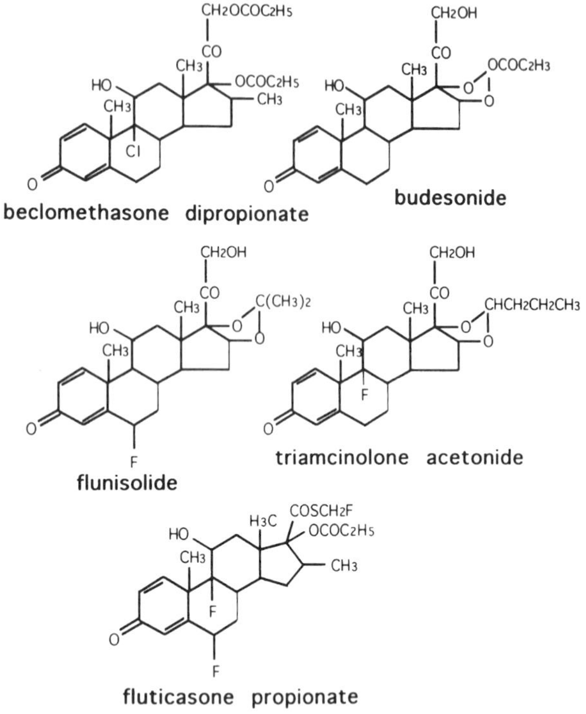

Figure 5-3. Chemical Structure of Topical Glucocorticoids Used for the Treatment of Asthma and Rhinitis.

prednisolone is a 16-17 carbon acetal substitution. Halogenation increases overall activity without specifically increasing topical effects. Also, budesonide is metabolized in the liver, but not in lung or skin tissue. These features may result in the favorable topical-to-systemic potency ratio for budesonide (Table 5-2). Fluticasone, likewise, has a high topical-to-systemic potency ratio.

THE GLUCOCORTICOID RECEPTOR

The glucocorticoid receptor has been purified, cloned, and sequenced and remains one of the most widely studied and best characterized of the steroid receptors. Non-protein-bound glucocorticoids, to which the glucocorticoid receptor is eventually bound, are thought to enter the cell via passive diffusion through the plasma membrane. A number of steps are required before the

Table 5-2. Relative Topical and Systemic Potencies of Topical Glucocorticoids

Glucocorticoid	Relative topical potency	Relative systemic potency	Topical–systemic potency ratio
Budesonide	1.0	1.0	1.0
Beclomethasone dipropionate	0.4	3.5	0.1
Flunisolide	0.7	12.8	0.05
Triamcinolone acetonide	0.3	5.3	0.05
Fluticasone propionate	1.7	0.07	25

Source Brattsand R, Thalen A, Roempke K, Gruvstad E. Development of new glucocorticosteroids with a very high ratio between topical and systemic activities. Eur J Respir Dis 1982; 63(suppl 122):62–73.

corticosteroid binds to the glucocorticoid receptor and exerts its biological effects on target tissues.

The glucocorticoid receptor is known to exist in at least two affinity states. The unactivated receptor is a 9S complex of ~300kDa, while the activated receptor has a sedimentation coefficient of ~4S with a molecular mass of ~90kDa. The difference between the two forms is that the activated receptor is bound to two 90-kDa proteins, with one 56–59-kDa protein bound to the 90-kDa proteins. These proteins are from the family of proteins known as heat shock proteins (hsp), which are elicited by various stressors.

The first step involved in hormone binding appears to be phosphorylation of the soluble receptor in the cytoplasm of target cells, which may be required for binding and activation of the hormone-receptor complex. Following phosphorylation, the receptor binds to its two hsp90 proteins with subsequent binding of one hsp56 protein to the hsp90 proteins. Once bound to these proteins, the receptor complex is now able to bind to hormones. It is thought that binding to hsp90 stabilizes the receptor complex in the high affinity state for glucocorticoids. Interestingly, the glucocorticoid receptor is thought to bind to the various glucocorticoids in proportion to their intrinsic activities. Also, the number of receptors present is thought to correlate with the response to treatment.

Prior to translocation to the nucleus, where glucocorticoids exert their biological effects, the hormone-receptor complex must be activated or transformed. Activation is thought to be due to a conformational change resulting from a change in the charge of the receptor. The hormone-receptor complex dissociates from the hsps at his point. Translocation of the activated hormone-receptor complex to the nucleus is necessary for DNA binding and exertion of the biological effects of glucocorticoids. It is thought that heat stress can promote translocation of the unliganded or non-hormone-bound receptor to the nucleus.

The glucocorticoid receptor is regulated by a number of endogenous factors, which can affect hormone binding, activation, stabilization, degradation, and transcription activation of the receptor.

CELLULAR EFFECTS OF GLUCOCORTICOIDS

Glucocorticoids have effects on almost all cells that contribute to the inflammatory process, including lymphocytes, eosinophils, neutrophils, macrophages, monocytes, mast cells, and basophils (Table 5-3). Unfortunately, much of the information known regarding these effects comes from in vitro studies, with glucocorticoid concentrations and conditions that often do not represent physiologic concentrations obtained with conventional therapy.

Lymphocytes

While the importance of lymphocytes to the pathogenesis of asthma and allergic diseases remains unclear, there is evidence supporting their role in the induction of IgE-dependent responses and regulation of inflammatory responses. The effect of administration of glucocorticoids on lymphocytes is a modest reduction of the number of cells present in the circulation, with $CD4^+$ cells being affected to a greater degree than $CD8^+$ cells. The mechanism is not direct killing of the cells, but induction of a programmed cell death, or *apoptosis*, which occurs in a select population of lymphocytes. Short-term effects may also be related to a redistribution of cells.

Glucocorticoids also have a number of effects on lymphocyte function. These include inhibition of interleukin-2 production and inhibition of interleukin-2 receptor generation. Glucocorticoids are also widely known to inhibit antigen-driven lymphocyte proliferation. Glucocorticoids suppress antigen-stimulated production of

Table 5-3.   Cellular Effects of Glucocorticoids

Cells affected	Effects of glucocorticoids
Lymphocytes	Reduction of circulating cell numbers, apoptosis
	Inhibition of IL-2 production
	Inhibition of IL-2 receptor generation
	Inhibition of antigen-driven proliferation
	Inhibition of IL-4 production
Eosinophils	Reduction of circulating cell counts
	Reduction of epithelial and mucosal cell counts
	Reduction of cell influx into cutaneous late-phase response
	Inhibition of IL-4-and IL-5-mediated cell survival
Neutrophils	Reduction of cell influx into cutaneous late-phase response
	Reduction of cell influx after nasal challenge
Macrophages	Inhibition of IL-1 release
	Inhibition of interferon-γ release
	Inhibition of tumor necrosis factor release
	Inhibition of granulocyte-monocyte colony stimulating factor release
	Inhibition of enzyme release
Monocytes	Reduction of circulating cell counts
Mast cells	Reduction of mast cell–derived mediators after nasal challenge
	Possible reduction of histamine content and releasability
Basophils	Reduction of circulating cell counts
	Reduction of cell influx in cutaneous late-phase response

interleukin-4 by human lymphocytes. Interleukin-4 is the T-cell–derived cytokine known to stimulate proliferation of resting B cells and the immunoglobulin switch from IgM to IgE, upregulate IgE receptors, and act as activating factor for macrophages and neutrophils and a growth factor for T-cells.

Eosinophils

Eosinophils in peripheral blood and bronchoalveolar lavage fluid have been correlated to the severity of asthma. After systemic administration of glucocorticoids, circulating eosinophil counts are reduced. The mechanism for eosinophil margination is unknown, as is the site of eosinophil compartmentalization. It is known that this eosinopenic response is blunted in steroid-resistant asthmatics, those patients who do not appear to respond to conventional high-dose systemic glucocorticoid therapy. After inhaled administration, epithelial and mucosal eosinophils are reduced, correlating with improvement of symptoms. Glucocorticoids inhibit the influx of eosinophils in the cutaneous late-phase response. Glucocorticoids also inhibit interleukin-4- and interleukin-5-mediated eosinophil survival.

Neutrophils

While the role of neutrophils in the pathogenesis of asthma and rhinitis remains unclear, in allergen challenge models of the airways and skin, the influx of neutrophils has been observed. The response of circulating neutrophils to glucocorticoids is increased by two- to four-fold after a single dose, as opposed to being reduced as noted with other inflammatory cells.

Although the influx of neutrophils into cutaneous late-phase reactions may be inhibited by oral glucocorticoid treatment, not all studies have supported this. Neutrophil influx after nasal challenge, however, is inhibited by topical glucocorticoid treatment.

Monocytes and macrophages

High numbers of macrophages are found in bronchoalveolar lavage fluid of allergic asthmatics, with activation present after antigen challenge. Glucocorticoids reduce the numbers of tissue macrophages in skin, and inhibit their release of interleukin-1, interferon-γ, tumor necrosis factor, granulocyte-monocyte colony stimulating factor, and various enzymes. Glucocorticoids also reduce the number of circulating monocytes.

Mast cells

Mast cells are well known to be associated with the allergic response. In asthma, mast cells are present in increased numbers and have increased releasability for their granules either spontaneously or via increased sensitivity to anti-IgE stimulation, which results in a lower threshold for the release of histamine as compared to nonasthmatic subjects. Asthmatic airways also appear to have an increased sensitivity to mast cell–derived bronchospastic mediators such as histamine, prostaglandin D2, and leukotriene C4.

Glucocorticoids have limited direct effects on mast cells. Treatment with glucocorticoids has no effect on the release of mast cell–derived mediators after antigen exposure. Glucocorticoids do not inhibit the release of histamine and leukotrienes from cultured human mast cells from various tissues. Topical glucocorticoid treatment prevents the appearance of mast cell mediators following nasal antigen challenge; however, biopsy data have shown little or no difference in the number of mast cells present when compared to normal. The effects of glucocorticoid treatment on the histamine-releasing ability of mast cells vary. Data from nasal biopsies suggest that histamine content and the proportion of histamine released are reduced by glucocorticoids, while data from nasal scrapings suggest an effect on histamine content only. In asthmatic subjects, a significant reduction of mast cells in the epithelium and mucosa after inhaled glucocorticoid treatment has been observed. No effects on degranulation were noted, however. Much of the effects of glucocorticoids on mast cells are likely due to their effect on the release of mast cell growth factors (interleukin-3, interleukin-4, granulocyte-monocyte colony stimulating factor) from other cell types.

Basophils

Increased numbers of basophils have been observed in late reactions in skin and airways. Also, the release of histamine in the late reaction is considered basophil derived. Glucocorticoids inhibit the influx of basophils and the late, but not immediate, appearance of histamine in the cutaneous late-phase response. Glucocorticoids also significantly reduce the numbers of circulating basophils.

EFFECTS ON CELL TRAFFICKING AND CHEMOTAXIS

A number of effects of glucocorticoids on cell trafficking and chemotaxis have been observed. Glucocorticoids reduce the influx of basophils and eosinophils in the cutaneous late-phase response to allergen challenge. Dexamethasone also inhibits the production of monocyte chemotactic-activating factor (MCAF) by human fibrosarcoma cells stimulated with interleukin-1 and tumor necrosis factor.

EFFECTS ON MEDIATOR SYNTHESIS AND RELEASE

Glucocorticoids block numerous mediators involved in the inflammatory process, including prostaglandins, leukotrienes, thromboxanes, and other arachidonic acid metabolites, as well as histamine, bradykinin, and the cytokines interleukin-1, interleukin-2, tumor necrosis factor, and interferon-γ. Topical glucocorticoid treatment reduces the amount of histamine releasing factors, cytokines produced by lymphocytes, monocytes, macrophages, platelet, and neutrophils, in nasal washings of patients with allergic rhinitis. While the molecular mechanisms for these actions are similar in terms of their dose-response relationships, steroid specificity, and requirement of RNA and protein synthesis, the cellular mechanisms vary. For example, T-cell synthesis of interferon-γ, granulocyte-monocyte colony stimulating factor, and interleukin-3 may be blocked at the level of transcription. Synthesis of interleukin-1 and tumor necrosis factor appears to be blocked at both the transcription and translation levels.

EFFECTS ON VASCULAR PERMEABILITY

Glucocorticoids inhibit the production and release of various mediators that are implicated as causing or potentiating microvascular leakage. Glucocorticoids inhibit the production of prostaglandins in vivo, thereby reducing their effects. Glucocorticoids also inhibit phospholipase A2, which reduces arachidonic acid release and subsequent formation of leukotrienes and PAF. The effects of glucocorticoids on histamine, a mediator important in vascular permeability, have been variable. However, release of histamine from basophils has been reduced with glucocorticoid treatment.

EFFECTS ON β-ADRENERGIC RECEPTOR ACTIVITY

Glucocorticoids are apparently necessary for normal β-adrenoceptor function. Without glucocorticoids, the threshold for receptor stimulation increases significantly. Glucocorticoids also potentiate the bronchodilatory effects of β-adrenergic agonists.

Tachyphylaxis to β-adrenergic agonists has been a long-standing topic of research. A number of studies have demonstrated that the reduced β-adrenergic response observed in cells from asthmatic patients is due to prolonged exposure to β-adrenergic agonist agents. The development of tachyphylaxis, demonstrated in normal and asthmatic subjects following administration of β-adrenergic agents, is possibly due to a reduction in β_2-adrenergic receptors on leukocytes. Treatment with glucocorticoids reverses this process. One study found that the peak effect of tachyphylaxis occurs over a short period (four weeks) after four times daily dosing and appears to influence the duration of action more than the peak bronchodilatory effect of albuterol. In this study, isoproterenol was also examined; however, no tachyphylaxis was observed. It remains unclear whether tachyphylaxis plays a clinically important role in the severity of asthma and whether glucocorticoids prevent β-adrenergic-induced desensitization.

EFFECTS ON BRONCHIAL HYPERREACTIVITY

Glucocorticoid therapy, especially inhaled administration, has the beneficial effect of reducing bronchial hyperreactivity in the treatment of asthma with prolonged treatment. This is presumably due to the anti-inflammatory effects of the glucocorticoids. Recent studies have demonstrated that budesonide and beclomethasone dipropionate reduced asthma symptoms as well as bronchial hyperreactivity in adults and children. Beneficial effects on bronchial hyperreactivity have been observed in as little as three weeks, and with long-term treatment no plateau has been observed with up to 22 months of treatment. Unfortunately, discontinuation of the inhaled glucocorticoid has often been shown to result in a disappearance of the beneficial effects within a few weeks to a few months.

PHARMACOKINETICS

The magnitude and duration of effect of glucocorticoids not only depend on the binding of glucocorticoids to the receptor and susceptibility of the target tissues, but also relate to the tissue concentrations resulting from the dose and frequency of dosing and the absorption, distribution, and elimination of glucocorticoids from the body. These can have profound influences on dosing strategies.

Absorption

Orally administered glucocorticoids must first be absorbed to cause any localized activity in the lung. Drug absorption can be affected by gastrointestinal transit time, permeability of the gastrointestinal mucosa, pH, and mucus content. Because of their lipophilicity, glucocorticoids are readily absorbed from the gastrointestinal tract and tissues. In general, the absorption of glucocorticoids is not affected by age, disease state, or smoking. Alternatively, antacid therapy may reduce prednisolone bioavailability. Relative bioavailability after antacids has been described as being 57 to 74% in normal patients, as compared to absorption without prior antacids, and 65 to 87% in patients with chronic active liver disease.

Only some initial delay in absorption with no effects on bioavailability has been reported in patients with inflammatory bowel disease.

Although limited data are available regarding systemic absorption of topically administered (intranasal and orally inhaled) glucocorticoids, there is evidence that these are absorbed systemically to some degree. Plasma concentrations are measurable after inhaled administration of as little as $400\,\mu g$ of triamcinolone acetonide, and may also be detectable for other inhaled glucocorticoids with comparable doses.

Distribution

Systemically active glucocorticoids are unique in that they undergo an interconversion reaction. For example, prednisone, which is inactive, must be converted to its active form, prednisolone. Reversible metabolism occurs rapidly in the liver and eventually reaches an equilibrium with prednisolone concentrations approximately ten-fold higher than prednisone concentrations when measured from the blood compartment. While this process has been reported to be impaired with acute viral hepatitis, chronic active hepatocellular disease, and hepatic cirrhosis, interconversion is not necessarily reduced with liver disease. Protein binding of prednisolone has been reported to be reduced with liver disease, resulting in increased serum concentrations of free prednisolone.

Clearance

The clearance of systemic glucocorticoids has been well characterized (Table 5-4). It has been shown that the rate of elimination is not usually affected by asthma. The potential for hepatic diseases to

Table 5-4. Pharmacokinetic Parameters of Systemic Glucocorticoids

Glucocorticoid	Clearance (ml/minute)	Half-life (minutes)	Serum protein binding (%)
Hydrocortisone	230	90–120	90
Dexamethasone	200	240	unknown
Methylprednisolone	400	150	unknown
Prednisolone	125	150–210	85–90

SOURCE: Ellul-Micallef R. Pharmacokinetics and pharmacodynamics of glucocorticosteroids. In: Jenne JW, Murphy S, eds. Drug therapy for asthma. Research and clinical practice. New York: Marcel Dekker, 1987:463–516.

reduce glucocorticoid clearance is well established. Liver disease is not, however, a significant factor in individualizing doses since prednisolone is extensively metabolized in other body organs. A number of concomitant medications can alter glucocorticoid clearance, either reducing or enhancing elimination (Table 5-5). Most notable are the anticonvulsants phenytoin, phenobarbital, and carbamazepine, which can result in an increased rate of elimination for dexamethasone, prednisolone, and methylprednisolone. While methylprednisolone appears to be affected to a greater degree than prednisolone, clearance of both prednisolone and methylprednisolone can be enhanced. Prednisolone clearance has been increased by 41%, 79%, and 76% and methylprednisolone clearance has been increased by 208%, 341%, and 478% with concomitant phenobarbital, carbamazepine, and phenytoin, respectively. In contrast, phenobarbital has resulted in an increase of dexamethasone clearance by 40%. Rifampin can also enhance the clearance of these glucocorticoids and result in a diminished therapeutic effect. A drug which can reduce prednisolone and methylprednisolone elimination is ketoconazole. Reductions of elimination by 27% and 60% have been described for prednisolone and methylprednisolone, respectively. Erythromycin and troleandomycin can also delay

Table 5-5. Major Drug Interactions with Systemic Glucocorticoids

Glucocorticoid affected	Interacting drug	Effect
Dexamethasone	Carbamazepine	Increased clearance
	Phenobarbital	Increased clearance
	Phenytoin	Increased clearance
Methylprednisolone	Carbamazepine	Increased clearance
	Phenobarbital	Increased clearance
	Phenytoin	Increased clearance
	Rifampin	Increased clearance
	Ketoconazole	Reduced clearance
	Troleandomycin	Reduced clearance
Prednisolone	Antacids	Reduced bioavailability
	Carbamazepine	Increased clearance
	Phenobarbital	Increased clearance
	Phenytoin	Increased clearance
	Rifampin	Increased clearance
	Ketoconazole	Reduced clearance
	Oral contraceptives	Reduced clearance

glucocorticoid clearance; however, studies have shown that this effect is limited to methylprednisolone. In general, a 70% reduction of methylprednisolone clearance can be expected with concomitant troleandomycin therapy. Oral contraceptives reduce prednisolone elimination by approximately one half. For the intranasal and inhaled glucocorticoids, there is no information regarding their disposition with concomitant medications.

PHARMACODYNAMICS

The duration of glucocorticoid effect, when measured by suppression of whole-blood histamine in humans, was demonstrated to be approximately the same for a regimen of methylprednisolone in a single dose of 40 mg and a split regimen of 20 mg followed by 5 mg eight hours later. These studies suggest that the frequency of dosing may be more important than the actual dose. This principle has been demonstrated in two studies with inhaled budesonide. When regimens of four times daily versus twice daily dosing of budesonide in the same total daily dose were compared, asthmatics were consistently better controlled on the four times daily regimens. Systemic effects, when measured by serum cortisol concentrations and circulating eosinophil counts, were not significantly different between the two regimens; however, trends for increased effects were seen with the four times daily regimen at the higher doses studied.

Studies on the dosing schedule of glucocorticoids, both inhaled and oral, have demonstrated that the timing of the doses can have a significant effect on asthma control. Two studies have demonstrated better asthma control with 3 P.M. dosing of oral glucocorticoids. One study specifically examined patients with nocturnal asthma and also demonstrated pronounced effects on the nocturnal influx of inflammatory cells. Adverse effects with such dosing regimens, however, require further study. An investigation of twice daily dosing regimens of inhaled budesonide administered at 8 A.M. and noon, or 8 A.M. and 8 P.M., demonstrated significantly reduced plasma cortisol and serum osteocalcin concentrations as compared with the morning-only regimen.

SUMMARY

Glucocorticoids have a number of actions on the many pathogenic mechanisms, including effects on inflammatory cell trafficking and chemotaxis and mediator synthesis and release. Effects are also observed on vascular permeability, β-adrenergic receptor activity, and bronchial hyperresponsiveness. These effects of glucocorticoids can be altered by a number of factors, including the route of delivery and concomitant medications. As the knowledge of the pathophysiologic and immunologic mechanisms for asthma and allergic rhinitis expands, opportunities will present themselves to understand the benefits and limitations of glucocorticoid therapy. This should lead to better insight into the design of treatment to optimize the effect of glucocorticoid therapy but also to recognize its shortcomings and to the design of improved glucocorticoids or better forms of alternative treatment.

II. CLINICAL USE OF GLUCOCORTICOIDS IN ASTHMA

CHRONIC ASTHMA

The use of corticosteroids in chronic asthma depends on the severity of the illness. Currently chronic asthma can be classified as mild, moderate, or severe, depending on symptoms and level of pulmonary function.

Mild asthma

Mild asthma is defined as asthma with brief, intermittent symptoms (attacks less often than once or twice a week, and with nocturnal symptoms occurring less often than twice a month). Patients are asymptomatic between symptomatic periods and have baseline peak expiratory flow rate (PEFR) greater than 80% of predicted. There is usually less than 20% variability in PEFR. In both adults and children, inhaled corticosteroids are not currently recommended, but rather intermediate-acting β-agonists are the usual treatment of choice (Figure 5-4). However, because of the concern for the development of long-term sequelae of chronic asthma such as subepithelial fibrosis due to ongoing airway inflammation, studies are now under way to determine whether early institution of inhaled steroids in mild asthma is warranted.

Moderate asthma

Moderate asthma is defined by symptomatic episodes occurring more than once or twice a week, with nocturnal awakenings more than twice a month and symptoms requiring up to daily use of an intermediate-acting β_2-agonist. Peak expiratory flow rates range

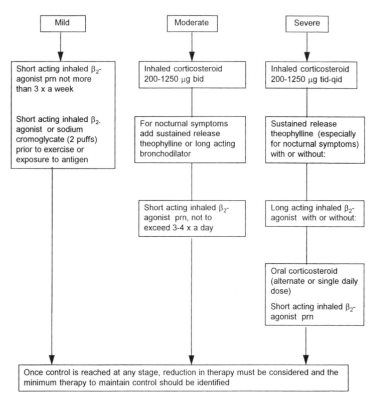

Figure 5-4. Recommendations for the use of corticosteroids in the management of chronic asthma in adults. Abbreviations: prn = as needed; qid = 4 times daily; tid = 3 times daily. SOURCE: McGill KA, Joseph B, Busse WW. Corticosteroids in the treatment of asthma. Practical recommendations. Clin Immunother 1995;4:16–48, with permission.

from 60 to 80% of that predicted at baseline, with a variability of 20 to 30%. For adults, this stage of asthma is frequently managed by the use of an inhaled steroid on a long-term basis for control of airway inflammation (see Figure 5-4). Further symptom control may require a long-acting β-agonist bronchodilator by inhalation or consideration of a sustained theophylline preparation. In addition, intermittent symptoms may be managed by an intermediate-acting inhaled β₂-agonist.

In children, sodium cromoglycate or nedocromil is usually the anti-inflammatory agent of choice. However, if symptoms are not adequately controlled by these therapies, institution of inhaled steroids may be necessary (Figure 5-5).

Dosing recommendations for use of inhaled corticosteroids in the treatment of asthma in adults can be found in Table 5-6. Optimal dosing depends on the severity of the patient's illness and needs to be evaluated periodically for either "step up" or "step down" modification. Similarly, in children, dosage recommendations depend on the severity of the child's asthma (Figure 5-6). On occasion, higher doses of inhaled glucocorticoids may be used in order to avoid prolonged use of oral corticosteroid therapy.

Severe asthma

Patients with severe asthma have frequent exacerbations of symptoms and recurrent episodes of nocturnal awakening and are unable to perform routine physical activities. The peak expiratory flow

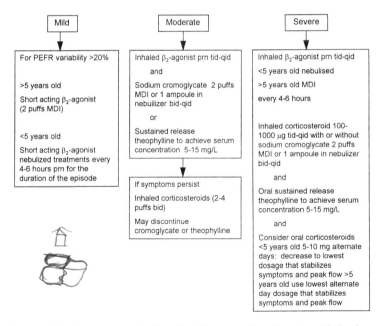

Figure 5-5. Recommendations for the use of corticosteroids in the management of chronic asthma in children. Abbreviations: bid = twice daily; MDI = metered-dose inhaler; PEFR = peak expiratory flow rate; prn = as needed; qid = 4 times daily; tid = 3 times daily. SOURCE: McGill KA, Joseph B, Busse WW. Corticosteroids in the treatment of asthma. Practical recommendations. Clin Immunother 1995; 4:16–48, with permission.

Table 5-6. Dosage Recommendations for Inhaled Corticosteroids in the Treatment of Adults with Asthma

Corticosteroid[a]	Dosage form (µg/actuation)		Dosage recommendation (µg/day)		
	MDI[b]	DPI[c]	Low dosage[d]	Moderate dosage[e]	High dosage[f]
Beclomethasone dipropionate	42, 50, 100, 200, 250	100, 200, 400	200–600	600–1000	>1000
Budesonide	50, 200	100, 200, 400	200–800	800–1600	>1600
Flunisolide	250		500–1000	1000–2000	>2000
Fluticasone propionate	25, 50, 125, 250	50, 100, 250, 500	100–750	750–1500	>1500
Triamcinolone acetonide	100		400–800	800–1600	>1600

[a] Availability varies among markets.

[b] MDI = metered-dose inhaler.

[c] DPI = dry powder inhaler.

[d] Indicated when symptoms interfere with daily activities; use of a β-agonist inhaler 2 to 4 times/day; small variations in peak expiratory flow rate (PEFR).

[e] Indicated when more severe symptoms >1 to 2 times/week; exacerbations affecting sleep and activity levels; occasional emergency care; use of a β-agonist >4 times/day.

[f] Indicated when frequent/continual symptoms, or nighttime or early awakenings; use of a β-agonist inhaler >4 times/day; FEV₁ and PEFR 60 to 85% of predicted; PEFR variability >30%.

SOURCE: McGill KA, Joseph B, Busse WW. Corticosteroids in the treatment of asthma. Practical recommendations. Clin Immunother 1995;4:16–48, with permission.

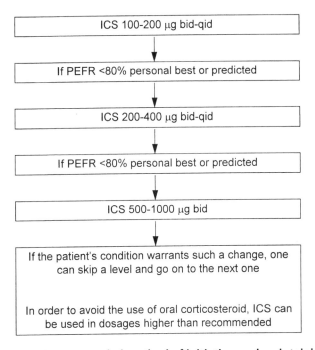

Figure 5-6. Recommended method of initiating and maintaining a child on inhaled corticosteroids. Abbreviations: bid = twice daily; ICS = inhaled corticosteroids; PEFR = peak expiratory flow rate; qid = 4 times daily. SOURCE: McGill KA, Joseph BA, Busse WW. Corticosteroids in the treatment of asthma. Practical recommendations. Clin Immunother 1995;4:16–48, with permission.

rate is less than 60% of predicted with variability greater than 30% and bronchodilator therapy may not return the PEFR to normal levels. Such patients often continue to have symptoms in spite of high-dose inhaled corticosteroids and supportive bronchodilator therapy. Such patients may require oral corticosteroids on a chronic basis, either on an alternate-day or single daily dose. The desired approach is to maintain the patient on the minimum dose of oral steroids required to control asthma symptoms and to minimize adverse systemic effects. Often, high doses of inhaled corticosteroids are initiated (1000 to 2000 μg per day) in addition to oral corticosteroids, with the intent of reducing the dosage of oral steroids over time. The ability to withdraw oral corticosteroids will depend on the severity of the disease. The intent of treatment is to withdraw the patient from the oral corticosteroids entirely, but this may not be possible. Doses of oral steroids can be reduced every one or two weeks by 1 to 5 mg per day, depending on the initial starting dose. Ideally, once-a-day dosing or alternate-day therapy should be employed where possible. Relief of nighttime symptoms may be achieved by administering the dose between 3 and 5 p.m In some refractory patients, administration of oral corticosteroids in divided doses may be necessary. The general principle is applied to both adults (see Figure 5-4) and children (see Figure 5-5). Patients experiencing acute exacerbations of their asthma may require increased doses of oral corticosteroids.

Acute asthma

Patients who experience acute exacerbations of their asthma may require short courses of oral corticosteroids over the course of three days to two weeks. The exact dose or duration of therapy of oral corticosteroids has not been consistently established, and various regimens based on empiric observations of physicians have been utilized. In general the dosage of prednisone for children is approximately 1 to 2 mg/kg per day with a maximum dose of 50 to 60 mg per day. In adults 30 to 80 mg per day is typical. A two- to three-times daily regimen of divided doses, in some instances, may be more effective than a single daily dose during acute exacerbations. Figure 5-7 gives a typical recommendation for the use of corticosteroids in the management of acute adults in asthma. An initial dose of 10 to 20 mg three times daily for one week followed by 10 to 30 mg daily for another week is not uncommon. If the patient's PEFR has increased to greater than 80% of baseline after seven days of therapy, the dose can be terminated without further tapering. If symptoms are prolonged, further tapering may be necessary and a longer course at a lower dose for one week followed by tapering may be necessary. If the corticosteroid dose is used for brief periods, tapering is not essential since adrenal suppression may recover quickly. However, rapid taper or abrupt withdrawal may cause the asthma to recur. Should short courses of oral corticosteroids fail to improve the patient with acute exacerbations, hospitalization or emergency room treatment may be necessary. Details regarding the dosages and administration of corticosteroids for such occurrences are contained in the chapter on the treatment of acute asthma. In children, an initial dose of prednisone for acute exacerbations is approximately 1 to 2 mg/kg per day administered in divided doses for approximately one week followed by 0.5 to 1 mg/kg per day as a single dose for another week (Figure 5-8). Children should be assessed after three to five

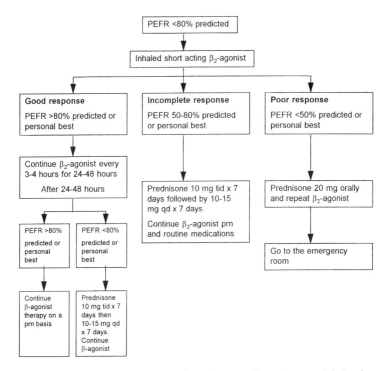

Figure 5-7. Recommendations for the use of corticosteroids in the management of acute asthma in an adult. Abbreviations: PEFR = peak expiratory flow rate; prn = as needed; qd = every day; tid = 3 times daily. SOURCE: McGill KA, Joseph B, Busse WW. Corticosteroids in the treatment of asthma. Practical recommendations. Clin Immunother 1995;4:16–48, with permission.

days to determine whether or not corticosteroids can be discontinued. If improvement of the PEFR to greater than 70% of predicted or personal best has occurred, the corticosteroids may be stopped. As with adults, if some improvement has occurred over the course of up to seven days, but complete improvement has not occurred, the dosage may be continued at the lower dose for a week until symptoms have improved or pulmonary functions have improved to 70 to 80% of predicted.

During the course of acute exacerbations, if the patient has been on inhaled steroids and inhaled corticosteroids and is tolerating them, they may be continued. For patients who have frequent acute exacerbations due to upper respiratory infections, a doubling of the dose of inhaled steroid may be instituted. If the patient fails

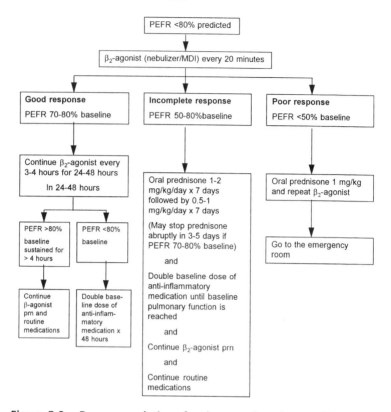

Figure 5-8. Recommendations for the use of corticosteroids in the management of acute asthma in children. Abbreviations: MDI = metered-dose inhaler; PEFR = peak expiratory flow rate. SOURCE: McGill KA, Joseph B, Busse WW. Corticosteroids in the treatment of asthma. Practical recommendations. Clin Immunother 1995;4: 16–48, with permission.

to respond to this increase in inhaled steroid dose over the course of 24 to 48 hours, oral corticosteroids are appropriate. Patients who have had frequent exacerbations requiring emergency room visits or hospitalization are candidates for short courses of oral corticosteroids, which may substantially reduce such morbidity.

Adverse effects of corticosteroids

Inhaled corticosteroids are advocated as maintenance therapy for moderate to severe asthma. Clearly, systemic absorption of the drugs occurs. However, the most significant adverse effects are localized to the upper respiratory tract primarily because of deposition in the oropharynx and larynx. Dysphonia is a common local adverse effect, occurring in 5 to 50% of patients. Often dysphonia can be alleviated by using spacer devices to eliminate deposition in the larynx. Rarely, dysphonia may be due to a local steroid myopathy. Oral candidiasis is an uncommon adverse effect of inhaled corticosteroids. With low doses of inhaled corticosteroids (less than 400 µg per day), candidiasis is uncommon, occurring in only about 5% of patients. Regular mouth rinsing and trial of spacer devices can often reduce the occurrence of candidiasis. In most instances, episodes are easily managed with topical antifungal agents to treat active infection. On occasion individuals may also experience cough and bronchospasm as a consequence of use of inhaled steroids; this may be due to the presence of oleic acid, which is a constituent of the suspension in some formulations. Changing to an alternative inhaled steroid may eliminate the problem, or the use of an intermediate-acting β-agonist prior to the inhaled corticosteroid may be helpful in preventing these side effects. Significant adrenal suppression with standard doses of inhaled corticosteroids appears to be rather unlikely. However, at high doses effects on adrenal function have been detected. The clinical significance of these is unclear. Nonetheless, since abnormalities in the HPA axis can occur, attempts should be made to reduce the dose to the smallest possible to achieve effective control of asthma. Growth suppression has been a concern in children using inhaled corticosteroids. One study of prepubescent boys receiving standard doses of inhaled corticosteroids (400 µg per day) noted a decrease in growth rate. However, in most studies, these children achieved full height potential. Cataract formation as a consequence of inhaled corticosteroids is extremely rare and in most instances is due to the concomitant use of oral corticosteroids. Even with high doses of inhaled corticosteroids, glucose metabolism does not appear to be substantially affected. In adults concerns regarding bone metabolism leading to osteoporosis have arisen. While dose-related effects have been shown in markers of skeletal metabolism such as serum osteocalcin levels, significant impairment of bone formation has not been clearly demonstrated.

The administration of oral corticosteroids on both a short-term and long-term basis does indeed have substantial side effects. In the short term, the major manifestations of orally administered corticosteroids include mood changes, appetite stimulation, fluid retention, alterations in glucose metabolism, and occasionally gastrointestinal effects including peptic ulceration. Aseptic necrosis of bone can occur even when oral corticosteroids are administered on a short-term basis.

The most profound systemic effects of long-term oral corticosteroids include cataract formation and osteoporosis as well as significant adrenal suppression, thinning of the skin, and excessive weight gain. Therefore, every opportunity should be made to withdraw long-term oral corticosteroids. Patients may be instructed in dietary management, avoidance of excessive sodium intake, and adequate calcium intake to help reduce the side effects.

In some instances alternative anti-inflammatory therapy can be considered, such as the use of methotrexate, cyclosporin, or other agents that may reduce the requirement for long-term systemic steroid therapy.

SUMMARY

Inhaled corticosteroids form the basis of the long-term therapy for moderate to severe asthma. Consideration of early institution in mild asthma is under way. Appropriate use of oral corticosteroids for acute exacerbations is extremely helpful in reducing the morbidity and possibly the mortality of asthma. Physicians should not hesitate to use such treatments when they are indicated.

SELECTED REFERENCES

Barnes PJ. Inhaled glucocorticoids for asthma. N Engl J Med 1995;332:868–875.

Dukes MNG, Holgate ST, Pauwels RA. Report of an international workshop on risk and safety of asthma therapy. Clin Exp Allergy 1994;24:160–165.

International Census Report on the diagnosis and treatment of asthma. Eur Respir J 1992;5:601–641.

McGill KA, Joseph B, Busse WW. Corticosteroids in the treatment of asthma. Practical recommendations. Clin Immunother 1995;4:16–48.

Reed CE. Glucocorticoids in asthma. Immunol Allergy Clin North Am 1993;13:903–915.

New Drugs for Asthma

6

There are currently five classes of antiasthmatic drugs in widespread use (Table 6-1). All these groups of drugs have been in use for ten years or more. A sixth class, leukotriene receptor antagonists, has recently been introduced into clinical practice. Although there have been changes in the prescribing of these drugs (earlier use of inhaled corticosteroids, changes in delivery systems with greater use of dry powder delivery systems and spacer devices for metered-dose inhalers), only the new class of leukotriene receptor antagonists has been introduced. With the improvements in understanding the basic mechanisms of asthma, new opportunities for developing antiasthmatic drugs have been discovered. Many of these new types of drugs have been studied in humans, and it is likely that in the next decade some of them will enter routine clinical practice.

When developing new antiasthmatic drugs, two basic approaches can be taken. One can either attempt to improve on currently available drugs by improving their efficacy or decreasing their side effects, or develop totally novel approaches.

MODIFICATION OF EXISTING ANTIASTHMATIC DRUGS

β_2-Agonists

β_2-agonists remain one of the cornerstones of antiasthmatic therapy. The most widely used short-acting β_2-agonists, salbutamol and terbutaline, however, suffer the disadvantage of a short duration of action of hours when given by inhalation. This has led to the development of long-acting β_2-agonists such as salmeterol and formoterol. These drugs have a duration of action of at least 12

Table 6-1. Current Classes of Antiasthmatic Drugs

β_2-agonists
Anticholinergics
Methylxanthines
Cromones
Corticosteroids
Leukotriene receptor antagonists

hours when given by inhalation and can improve disease control in mild and moderately severe asthma with an improvement in lung function. Some evidence from animal studies suggests that salmeterol has some anti-inflammatory properties in addition to its bronchodilatory effect. Investigation in man has not confirmed this anti-inflammatory effect. Both salmeterol and formoterol can block the late response to antigen challenge, and salmeterol can attenuate the increase in bronchial hyperresponsiveness seen after the late response. However, these effects may be due solely to function antagonism. Studies of biopsies from asthmatic patients treated with salmeterol for six weeks have failed to demonstrate any decrease in inflammation.

Although there is no evidence that tachyphylaxis occurs to the smooth muscle relaxant effects of salmeterol, recent work has suggested that some other effects of β_2-agonists, such as mast cell stabilization and prevention of induced bronchoconstriction, may demonstrate tachyphylaxis after prolonged administration. Whether this effect is of clinical relevance requires further evaluation.

Anticholinergics

Anticholinergic drugs are of some use in asthma, particularly in severe acute asthma. There is also some evidence that they may be of benefit in nocturnal asthma. Longer-acting inhaled anticholinergic drugs, such as oxitropium bromide, have been synthesized, and these may have advantages over the shorter-acting ipratropium bromide. More selective muscarinic antagonists are also being developed. The muscarinic receptor is thought to exist in at least five subtypes, although in the airways, only M1, M2, and M3 receptors have been demonstrated. M3 receptors are present on airway smooth muscle, and stimulation of these causes bronchoconstriction. M2 receptors are present prejunctionally on parasympathetic nerves; stimulation of the M2 receptor inhibits acetylcholine release and therefore prevents bronchoconstriction. The M1 receptors are present on parasympathetic ganglia and may facilitate neurotransmission. Current anticholinergic drugs block all three receptor subtypes, including the potentially beneficial M2 receptor. M3 or M1/M3 selective anticholinergic drugs may have advantages over current anticholinergics and are currently being evaluated in humans.

Methylxanthines

Methylxanthines have a variety of actions that may be of relevance in asthma therapy. However, their poor therapeutic index and side effects limit their usefulness. Attention recently has refocused on their ability to block the enzyme phosphodiesterase (PDE) and thus increase intracellular cyclic 3′,5′-adenosine monophosphate (cAMP) and cyclic guanylic acid (GMP) levels. PDE exists in a number of isoenzymes (PDE I to V), which are located in different tissues and have different characteristics. If methylxanthines are having their major effect by blocking PDE, then the potential exists to develop selective PDE isoenzyme inhibitors, which may be of comparable or greater activity than current methylxanthines but without their side effects. The main isoenzymes are also present in inflammatory cells, such as mast cells, eosinophils, and macrophages. Thus, the possibility exists that a dual bronchodilator/anti-inflammatory drug could be developed. Early studies with selective isoenzyme inhibitors have shown some activity. The ultimate value of this approach will depend on whether PDE inhibition is, in fact, the major therapeutic action of methylxanthines and on whether side effects can be reduced by isoenzyme-selective drugs.

Cromones

Disodium cromoglycate (DSCG) has been used in the treatment of asthma for 20 years, and the related drug nedocromil sodium has been introduced more recently. While safe and, in the case of DSCG, particularly effective in children, their activity in adults and in more severe asthma has been disappointing. Part of the problem in developing more active drugs of this class is that their precise mode of action is not clear. Recently, inhaled furosemide—but not oral furosemide or inhaled bumetanide—has been shown to have a spectrum of activity in clinical models of asthma very similar to that of DSCG. Inhaled furosemide, like DSCG, blocks the indirect challenges of antigen, exercise, hypotonic saline, and metabisulfite while having no effect on the direct challenges such as metha-choline and prostaglandin $F_{2\alpha}$. Inhaled furosemide is currently be-ing evaluated for its effect in chronic asthma. It is possible that the mechanism of action of inhaled furosemide may shed light on the mechanism of action of DSCG and allow the rational design of more potent drugs with a related mode of action. A common link may be due to blockade of choline ion channels.

Corticosteroids

Inhaled corticosteroids are recognized as fundamental in the treat-ment of all but the mildest of adult asthma and are now used with an increasing number of children and at higher doses, particularly in adults. This has led to increased concern about the long-term systemic side effects of inhaled steroids. New inhaled steroids with a greater ratio of topical potency to systemic side effects are now being developed. Of these new inhaled steroids, fluticasone propi-onate (FP) has high topical activity but almost 100% first-pass metabolism in the liver; thus, the swallowed portion of the drug (80 to 90%) cannot exert any systemic activity, and only the portion absorbed from the lung can cause systemic side effects. FP has been extensively investigated and shows greater potency than beclomethasone dipropionate (BDP). It is likely that FP and other new inhaled steroids with greater safety margins will be of particu-lar use in children and adults on high-dose inhaled steroids.

This, together with their clinical efficacy, is likely to keep inhaled steroids at the forefront of asthma treatment over the next ten years. Even with currently available antiasthmatic drugs, there is still a significant minority of patients who require long-term oral steroids or short courses of steroids for acute exacerbations. Deflazacort is an orally active corticosteroid that has been claimed to have fewer systemic side effects, particularly on bone, than prednisolone at doses causing equivalent anti-inflammatory effects. The data indicating equivalent anti-inflammatory activity are lim-ited, and no studies in asthma have been performed.

NOVEL APPROACHES TO ASTHMA THERAPY

Increased understanding of the pathophysiology of asthma has led to new targets for drug development, and in many cases com-pounds have now been developed and tested in humans that interfere with these pathways. Other novel therapies have been suggested by evaluating the effect of currently available drugs used for other diseases, such as methotrexate, cyclosporin A (CsA), and gold (Table 6-2).

1. Potassium channel activators

Potassium (K^+) channels are present on smooth muscle, and activation of K^+ channels leads to relaxation. K^+ channel activators were originally developed as antihypertensive agents, but studies have now been performed of these drugs in asthma. K^+ channel activators relax human bronchial smooth muscle in vitro. When studied in man, cromakalin has no effect on baseline airway tone or induced bronchoconstriction but does protect against morning drops in pulmonary function in asthmatic patients. Unfortunately, the effect of these drugs on vascular smooth muscle causing flushing, headache, and postural hypotension has limited their usefulness. Newer drugs selective for airway smooth muscle have been developed, and it is possible that inhalation of these drugs will decrease their side effects. K^+ channels are present on some inflammatory cells, so K^+ channel activators may have additional anti-inflammatory properties. For K^+ channel activators to be of clinical use, the cardiovascular side effects will need to be overcome.

2. Calcium channel blockers

Alterations in calcium flux are important in activating airway smooth muscle and a number of inflammatory cells. Calcium antagonists, such as nifedipine and verapamil, developed for cardio-

---

Table 6-2. Novel Antiasthmatic Drugs

1. Potassium channel activators
2. Calcium channel blockers
3. Drugs affecting asthmatic mediators
   a. Histamine
   b. Platelet-activating factor (PAF)
   c. Leukotrienes
   d. Prostanoids and thromboxane
4. Immunomodulation/Immunosuppressants
   a. Methotrexate
   b. Gold
   c. Hydroxychloroquine
   d. Cyclosporin A
5. Adhesion blockers
6. New peptide agonists and antagonists

---

vascular indications, have been studied in asthma. The studies have shown no direct bronchodilatory action but minor effects on indirect challenges, such as antigen and cold air. These calcium antagonists affect voltage–dependent calcium channels. It now seems likely that receptor-operated calcium channels and intracellular mobilization of calcium are of greater importance in asthma. Drugs affecting these alternative calcium pathways are now being developed that offer the prospect of being both bronchodilators and anti–inflammatory agents.

3. Drugs affecting asthmatic mediators

a. **Histamine:** Histamine was the first asthmatic mediator to be discovered. It is released on immunological and nonimmunological challenge of mast cells and basophils. Histamine causes bronchoconstriction, and asthmatics are hyperresponsive to its effect. Potent H1 histamine antagonists attenuate the early response to antigen and bronchoconstriction caused by cold air, exercise, and hypotonic saline. Antihistamines cause bronchodilatation acutely, but chronic use leads to tachyphylaxis. Despite all this evidence for a role of histamine in asthma, antihistamines are of only trivial use in chronic asthma. The story of antihistamines indicates graphically the problems of developing antimediator drugs of benefit in chronic asthma. It is most unlikely that even more potent antihistamines will be of clinical benefit in chronic asthma.

b. **Platelet activating factor antagonists:** Platelet activating factor (PAF) is an inflammatory mediator with a variety of actions of relevance to the pathogenesis of asthma. PAF is released from a variety of inflammatory cells found within the lungs, including macrophages, eosinophils, neutrophils, and platelets. It acts to attract and activate a variety of cells, including eosinophils, neutrophils, and platelets. PAF causes bronchoconstriction, but interest was increased by the observations that a single inhalation of PAF by normal subjects not only caused bronchoconstriction but also increased bronchial hyperresponsiveness for up to two weeks, thus mimicking one of the cardinal features of asthma. This increase in bronchial hyperresponsiveness following PAF inhalation has been confirmed by some groups but not by others.

Three very potent and specific PAF antagonists, WEB-2086, MK-287, and UK-74,505, have been evaluated in man. It is striking that these PAF antagonists have very different molecular structures. WEB-2086 is a benzodiazepine derivative and UK-74,505 shares many structural similarities with calcium antagonists. All three of these very active PAF antagonists have now been investigated for their effects on the early and late response to antigen challenge; there has been no effect at all on the early or late response to inhaled antigen or the increase in bronchial hyperresponsiveness occurring after antigen challenge. Preliminary results in chronic asthma with WEB-2086 have shown no effect on the requirements for inhaled steroids over a 12-week period. The most likely reason for the inability of PAF antagonists to block antigen-induced bronchoconstriction or be effective in chronic asthma is that PAF is not an important mediator in asthma. However, other possibilities are that more than one PAF receptor is present in humans and that the currently available drugs do not block this, or that PAF is mainly operating intracellularly and the drugs are affecting only extracellular PAF responses.

c. Drugs affecting the 5-lipoxygenase pathway: There is a considerable body of evidence that products of the 5-lipoxygenase pathway, the cysteinyl leukotrienes LTC4, D4, and E4 and the dihydroxyacid LTB4, play a role in the pathophysiology of asthma. The cysteinyl leukotrienes are potent causes of bronchoconstriction and may in certain circumstances increase bronchial hyperresponsiveness, promote edema formation, and act as mucus secretagogues. Although the pathophysiological role of leukotriene B4 in man is less clearly defined, it may have potential importance in recruiting and activating inflammatory cells, particularly neutrophils and eosinophils. There is good evidence that leukotrienes are produced in the lung, in clinical models of asthma such as antigen challenge, and they are present in acute severe asthma attacks and in chronic asthma.

Following the discovery of the structures of slow-reacting substance of anaphylaxis (SRS-A), an enormous research effort was put into developing new cysteinyl leukotriene antagonists, which have entered clinical practice (e.g., zafirlukast), while a number of these are still undergoing clinical trials. LY171883 is an orally active cysteinyl leukotriene antagonist, which at a dose of 400 mg shifts the LTD4 dose response curve to the right by about five-fold and gives a slight but statistically significant protection against the early response on allergen challenge but has no effect on the late response. In addition, LY171883 was shown to have a small protective effect against cold air–induced bronchoconstriction.

LY1717881 was studied for its effect in chronic asthma in a group of mild asthmatics, controlled previously on oral theophyllines and a β_2-agonist. LY171883 given for six weeks caused a small improvement in pulmonary function. There was a trend towards a decrease in rescue bronchodilator use, which was significant only for the subgroup using more than 23 mg of metaproterenol per week. It is not clear whether this effect is due to the cysteinyl leukotriene antagonist effect of LY171883, as the drug is also a PDE inhibitor. These early oral acetophenone derivatives had gastrointestinal side effects, and this, together with their relatively low potency, has led them to being superseded by other classes of compounds.

The newer leukotriene antagonists are much more potent drugs. ICI 204219 is an indazoline and SK&F 104353 is a leukotriene D4 analogue. ICI 204219, when given orally, can shift the inhaled leukotriene D4 dose response curve between 40- and 100-fold to the right. This improved potency enables it to block about 80% of the early response to inhaled antigen and approximately 50% of the late response. ICI 204219 was also shown to attenuate the increase in bronchial hyperresponsiveness occurring after the late response, although it is not clear if this effect is due to a genuine effect on bronchial hyperresponsiveness or to improvement in airway function at the time when bronchial hyperresponsiveness was measured. MK 571 has also been shown to have a major protective effect against the early and late response to antigen challenge. Both drugs have also been shown to protect against cold air or exercise-induced bronchoconstriction. SK&F 104353 is of interest because it is given by the inhaled route. At the doses at which it has been used, it would appear to shift a leukotriene D4 dose response curve about ten-fold to the right. It would also attenuate the early and late response to inhaled allergen. All three drugs have been shown to bronchodilate wheezy asthmatics, though the effect has been with MK 571, showing 20% improvement in FEV_1 and ICI 204219 a 7% improvement. The difference in these responses is likely due to the different patient group studied, with MK 571 being investigated in a group of mild asthmatics and ICI 204219 in a group of older, moderately severe asthmatics taking inhaled corticosteroids. A surprising and unexpected observation in these studies was that the bronchodilator effect of cysteinyl leukotrienes was additive to that of albuterol. It suggests that leukotriene antagonists may be able to bronchodilate by a mechanism not available to β_2-agonists. There has been a preliminary report of the effect of MK 571 in chronic dosage that suggests that it is of benefit. SK&F 104153 has also been used to shed further light on the long-standing puzzle of aspirin-induced asthma. A single dose of SK&F 104153 has been shown to block the effects of lysine aspirin challenge in a group of aspirin-sensitive asthmatics, and treatment of this group of patients with an LT antagonist may be particularly appropriate.

The results of the various studies of leukotriene antagonists have been consistent in that the early and weak drugs showed small effects on the clinical models of asthma in which they were studied, whereas the newer and more potent drugs have shown major effects. Definitive studies of these drugs in chronic asthma are ongoing, but the results of the studies in models of asthma and the acute studies in wheezy asthmatics suggest that these drugs should have a beneficial effect in asthma. The early acetophenone derivatives had dose-limiting gastrointestinal side effects; however, the new drugs seem free of any major side effects, and at present there is no evidence that any major dose-limiting toxicity is attributable to leukotriene antagonism. It seems likely that LT antagonists work in the presence of inhaled steroids, and are additive in their bronchodilator effect to β_2-agonists. They will be a useful addition in therapy and useful in children where physicians may wish to avoid inhaled steroids. As yet, there is little evidence of any anti-inflammatory action, and it is unlikely they will supplant steroids.

Effective 5-lipoxygenase (5-LO) inhibitors have been developed. Zileuton is a redox agent, which acts by blocking the redox reaction involving the iron-containing moiety in 5-LO inhibitor. Zileuton has been shown to block approximately 50% of urinary $LTe4$ production following antigen challenge and to attenuate the early response to antigen in those subjects who had good blockade of leukotriene production. Zileuton provides partial protection against cold air–induced bronchoconstriction. It has been reported as improving lung function in mild chronic asthma. MK-886 has a novel mode of action. It blocks the activation of the 5-LO enzyme by a protein termed 5-LO activating protein (FLAP). In a study of antigen challenge, MK-886 had a small protective effect on the early response to antigen.

d. Drugs affecting the cyclo-oxygenase pathway: Prostaglandin $F_{2\alpha}$ and prostaglandin D2 are potent bronchoconstrictors to which asthmatics are hyperreactive. Further, inhaled prostaglandin $F_{2\alpha}$ and prostaglandin D2 increase bronchial hyperresponsiveness to other mediators, thus mimicking one of the cardinal features of asthma. It is now generally accepted that all of the bronchoconstrictor prostanoids operate in the human lung by binding to a common thromboxane receptor. Thus, blockage of the bronchoconstrictor effect on a variety of prostanoids can be achieved with a single thromboxane antagonist. A number of studies demonstrated that the major arachidonic acid metabolite released from human mast cells was prostaglandin D2. These observations lead to the possibility that thromboxane A2 receptor antagonists might be beneficial in asthma.

Potent thromboxane receptor antagonists have now become available, such as BAYU-3405. This drug has a significant effect on the dose response curve to inhaled PGD2 but is without effect in exercise-induced asthma. The disappointing effects of these drugs in models of asthma and the knowledge that cyclo-oxygenase inhibitors are generally ineffective in asthma make it unlikely that these drugs will have a significant effect in chronic asthma.

4. Immunosuppressants

With the establishment of the role of low-dose cytotoxic drugs acting as steroid-sparing agents in rheumatoid arthritis, a number of studies of immunosuppressants in asthma took place in the 1970s. The results of these studies were generally disappointing. The increasing evidence of the role of inflammation in the pathogenesis of asthma has led to a resurgence of interest in the use of immunosuppressants in asthma. A comparison of these agents is found in Table 6-3.

a. Methotrexate: The dihydrofolate reductase inhibitor methotrexate has an established role as a steroid-sparing agent in rheumatoid arthritis and is established as an effective therapy in psoriasis. An initial double-blind placebo-controlled crossover trial of the effect of methotrexate (15 mg per week) on oral steroid requirement in asthma demonstrated that oral prednisone requirement fell, while control of asthma was unaffected. Since then, a number of other trials have been reported with variable outcomes. One of these studies with more than 60 steroid-dependent asthmatics treated for 28 weeks evaluated the effectiveness of either methotrexate 15 mg per week or matching placebo. There was a 14% fall in oral steroid requirement in the placebo group but a significantly greater (50% fall) in prednisone dosage in the methotrexate-treated group. The pattern of the response is of interest. The placebo and

Table 6-3. Comparative Efficacy of Novel Therapies in Asthma

Medication	Protection allergen challenge	Reduction AHR	Oral steroid dose reduction	Biopsy
High-dose inhaled glucocorticoids	LAR	+++	+++	ND
Methotrexate	ND	−	++	ND
Gold	ND	++	++	ND
Hydroxychloroquine	ND	ND	+++	ND
Cyclosporin A	ND	ND	++	ND

+++, marked effect; ++, moderate or inconsistent effect; +, some effect; −, no effect; ND, no data available. AHR, airway hyperresponsiveness. Resolution of inflammation is assumed based on a significant reduction in airway hyperresponsiveness, significant oral steroid dose reduction, or biopsy proven reduction in inflammatory cells with chronic therapy.

Modified from: Szefler SJ, Leung DYM. Asthma management. Past, present and future. In: Szefler SJ, Leung DYM (eds.), Severe asthma: Pathogenesis and clinical management (Lenfant C, executive ed., Lung biology in health and disease, Vol 86), New York: Marcel Dekker, 1996, pp 537–557, with permission.

methotrexate-treated groups did not diverge in their steroid requirement until eight weeks into the study, and steroid requirement was still falling at the end in the methotrexate group. Disappointingly, once methotrexate had a number of undesirable side effects, including liver fibrosis. There are also reports of opportunistic pneumonias, particularly pneumocystic carinae pneumonia (PCP) occurring in patients with asthma treated with methotrexate. The place of methotrexate in the treatment of asthma remains unclear but is worthy of consideration in patients on oral steroids who are suffering side effects.

b. Gold: Gold has been used as a treatment in Japan for a number of years, but until recently there have been few controlled trials in asthma. An open study of oral gold (auranofin) suggested an improvement in symptoms and decrease in bronchial hyperresponsiveness and a decrease in oral steroid requirement. Recently, a carefully conducted study of the effects of oral gold in steroid-dependent asthmatics showed a small decrease in oral steroid requirement with a mean increase in FEV_1 of 6.4% at 26 weeks. It is not clear that a longer duration of treatment would have led to any further benefit. The exact site of action of gold is not clear, but at least part of its action is by interfering with T-lymphocyte function.

c. Hydroxychloroquine: Hydroxychloroquine has been shown to be a steroid-sparing agent in rheumatoid arthritis. A recent open study of hydroxychloroquine in steroid-dependent asthma reported an impressive fall in steroid requirements. A double-blind placebo-controlled trial is now underway in the United States.

d. Cyclosporin A: The rationale for investigating the effect of cyclosporin A (CsA) in asthma came from work on the pathogenesis of asthma suggesting the involvement of the activated T-lymphocyte. CsA is a cycloundeca peptide which has revolutionized the effectiveness of organ transplantation. The mode of action of CsA has until recently been considered to be primarily on the T-lymphocyte. It prevents the clonal proliferation of $CD4^+$ T-lymphocytes by preventing IL-2 and IL-2 receptor expression. Recently, studies have suggested that it may also prevent cytokine expression for other cells including mast cells, eosinophils, and basophils; however, its primary mode of action is still considered to be on the T-lymphocyte. In a group of severe steroid-dependent asthmatics treated over a 12-week period, low-dose CsA (5 mg/kg per day) has been shown to increase pulmonary function and decrease the number of exacerbations requiring a boost in prednisolone dosage. The effects of CsA are variable, with some patients showing no response and others very large improvements in pulmonary function. Another study did not show any benefit of CsA. CsA has a number of undesirable side effects, principally causing a decrease in renal function. However, over the course of the 12-week study, there was a mean 10% decrease in glomerular filtration and no other serious adverse events.

Although none of the immunosuppressant agents yet studied in asthma have the necessary specificity of action to be entirely confident as to their exact site of action, the evidence is suggestive that both CsA and gold affect T-lymphocyte function. While the currently available drugs are kept from widespread use by their toxicity, this area opens up possibilities for more specific and safe drugs to be developed, targeted either pharmacologically or by route of delivery. It is likely that developing drugs which act on the T-lymphocyte and cytokine axis will provide useful new therapies for asthma. As they are acting high up in the inflammatory cascade, they should have profound disease-modifying, anti-inflammatory actions. IL-5 is a prime candidate, and antagonists to this cytokine are undergoing investigation.

5. Adhesion blockers

Adhesion molecules are a recently identified target, which may allow manipulation by drugs. There are no studies in humans, but a study of an anti-ICAM-1 monoclonal antibody in a primate model shows activity against eosinophil accumulation after antigen challenge but no effect on chronic airway inflammation.

6. Neuropeptide agonists and antagonists

A variety of targets for drug development exist in the peptinergic nervous system. Drugs blocking bronchoconstrictor neuropeptides, such as neurokinin A and agonists acting at the bronchodilator VIP receptor, are being developed. Their value will depend on how important the peptinergic nervous system is in asthma and whether one dominant neuropeptide can be identified.

CONCLUSION

The huge increase in the understanding of basic pathophysiological mechanisms in asthma has opened up many novel therapeutic possibilities, and it is almost certain that some of these will enter clinical practice in the next few years. Improved inhaled steroids are likely to be an important development. Leukotriene antagonists are showing activity that suggests they will be safe, active, and attractive as add-on therapies in adults, and in children they may be of value in postponing the need for inhaled steroids. Leukotriene inhibitors will usher in a new class of antiasthmatic drugs. Safe oral or inhaled therapies that act high in the inflammatory cascade at the level of the lymphocyte/macrophage and their associated cytokines present the opportunity to develop new anti-inflammatory agents.

It has often been claimed that so many mediators and cells are present in the asthmatic response that a drug acting exclusively against one element is unlikely to be effective. As more novel therapies become available it can be seen that this gloomy prospect is not true. Some mediators are present but unimportant and probably play only a small role, leaving an enhanced role for other mediators. The new approaches to treating asthma will lead to a decreased role for older drugs and teach us more about asthma pathophysiology.

SELECTED REFERENCES

Chung KF. Leukotriene receptor antagonists and biosynthesis inhibitors: potential breakthrough in asthma therapy. Eur Respir J 1995;8:1203–1213.

Holliday SM, Faulds D, Sorkin EM. Inhaled fluticasone propionate. A review of its pharmacodynamic and pharmacokinetic properties, and therapeutic use in asthma. Drugs 1994;47:318–331.

Moss RB. Alternative pharmacotherapies for steroid-dependent asthma. Chest 1995;107;817–825.

Schudt C, Tenor H, Hatzelmann A. PDE isoenzymes as targets for anti-asthma drugs. Eur Respir J 1995;8:1179–1183.

Asthma in Children

7

Asthma is a leading cause of morbidity among children throughout the world. In the United States, asthma accounts for 2.2 million pediatrician visits per year and 38 million restricted activity days. Within the past 15 years, the prevalence of asthma has been increasing from 5.3% (1963 to 1965) to 7.6% (1986 to 1990) in children aged 6 to 11 years. This increase may be due to increasing urbanization, increasing pollution, more time spent indoors and/or more accurate diagnosis of asthma. Death rates have been increasing steadily in the last 20 years, to 6.2% per year. Hospitalizations have also increased steadily in the last ten years, especially in children aged four years or less, where rates are 4.8 per 1000. Hospitalizations are three times higher in blacks than in whites.

The median age of onset of asthma is four years, and more than 20% of children develop symptoms within the first year of life. Risk factors for early onset include atopy, especially early demonstration of positive skin tests to milk, eggs, and other foods. This risk factor is clearly genetic, in that the parental history is almost as strong a risk factor as an elevated level of IgE in cord blood. The association with parental smoking is much less clear, and most studies have shown a weak or insignificant association with the onset or severity of asthma. Other obvious risk factors for early onset include neonatal lung disease, reduced lung volume in otherwise healthy infants, and respiratory infections, especially with the respiratory syncytial virus. Forty to 50% of infants with RSV bronchiolitis develop chronic asthma. Allergen exposure is capable of altering asthma symptoms and increasing bronchial hyperresponsiveness.

Most asthmatics have acute obstructive responses to various precipitants, including viral respiratory infections, allergens, exercise, irritants, drugs, and weather changes. The association between respiratory virus infections and significant wheezing episodes in asthmatic patients is much clearer in children, where 60% of such infections are accompanied by wheezing, than it is in adults, where 20% of such infections are accompanied by wheezing.

EVALUATION

The NHLBI classification permits a simple categorization for therapeutic intervention, yet may not reflect the complexity of the disease:

Stage 1: comprises the early onset of symptoms and could be characterized by sudden, episodic exacerbations, usually precipitated by respiratory infections and occasionally by allergen exposure. Treatment is targeted to provide rapid relief of respiratory distress with β-adrenergic agonists. Short courses of oral glucocorticoids may be necessary for severe acute exacerbations.

Stage 2: the symptoms are more frequent and require daily therapy.

Stage 3: symptoms now significantly affect quality of life.

Stage 4: characterized by deteriorating pulmonary function, persistent symptoms, and frequent life-threatening episodes of acute exacerbations; may also exhibit severe hypoxic episodes.

The physician should consider the possibility of alternative diagnoses such as cystic fibrosis, immunodeficiency, gastroesophageal reflux, tracheal esophageal fistula, recurrent pneumonia, aspiration, or other rare disorders, such as congenital heart disease, pulmonary lobe sequestration, immotile cilia, and bronchiectasis. Appropriate laboratory tests, such as chest x-rays, and tests of arterial blood gases, sweat, immunoglobulins, and pulmonary function can be obtained, based on the level of suspicion, and are not indicated in every patient.

Patients requiring daily therapy must be educated about asthma care for themselves and their families. Laboratory evaluation should identify precipitants associated with asthma exacerbations and involve pulmonary function testing including daily peak flow monitoring. Allergy skin tests are indicated at this stage. Peak flow monitoring should be incorporated.

Treatment should be directed at eliminating environmental allergen exposure. Medication treatment should be designed to relieve symptoms that could minimize inflammation. Asthma education should cover the technique of administering medication, methods to treat acute exacerbations, and the importance of compliance with the treatment protocol.

Patients with asthma affecting quality of life frequently require systemic glucocorticoid therapy for acute exacerbations and may need it for maintenance therapy. These patients are often considered for high-dose inhaled steroid trials or other anti-inflammatory therapy (troleandomycin, methotrexate, gold, hydroxychloroquine, or dapsone).

Patients on long-term high-dose systemic steroid therapy need close review for adverse effects, including attentive physical examination for excessive steroid exposure, growth suppression, myopathy, hypertension, cataracts, weight gain, central obesity, and easy bruising, as well as laboratory tests such as bone densitometry, 24-hour urinary free cortisol, and calcium excretion.

Patients classified as Stage 4 are at risk for asthma mortality and for disabling complications from their severe lung disease. These patients require special care and consideration for more aggressive forms of immunomodulator therapy.

For patients who are poorly responsive to glucocorticoid therapy, especially those with minimal adverse effects, measurements of steroid pharmacokinetics, specifically absorption and elimination, can provide useful information.

MANAGEMENT

Environment

Allergen avoidance is an essential first step in treating allergic asthma:

House dust mites: House dust mite allergy is caused by pyroglyph mites, which infest bedding, rugs, and other fabrics. Close exposure such as sleeping in an infested bed or lying on an infested rug is important for sensitization and induction of inflammation and symptoms. To avoid mite allergen, one should install airtight covers completely covering the mattress and pillow. Mites in bedding can be removed by washing in hot water (55°C) or by dry cleaning: infestation usually recurs within a few weeks.

Furry pets: Pets contribute their own potent allergens, and approximately a third of children with asthma have positive skin tests to cat or dog. The only rational solution is to eliminate the pet from a household with a sensitized child. Alternatively allergen can be reduced by washing the pet every one to two weeks, although this is not fully established.

Molds: Mold antigens are ubiquitous in a home environment, and more than 25% of asthmatic children have positive skin tests. In general, the problem is worse in older houses and in moist environments. The most effective way of removing mold and mildew is to remove contaminated materials and to attempt to reduce home moisture content.

Cockroaches: Cockroaches also contribute important allergens in urban environments, especially in the Middle Atlantic and Southeastern states. Elimination of the antigen usually requires pest control consultation and careful clean-up of the remaining insect parts and feces, which can be very widespread and contain high concentrations of antigen.

Tobacco smoke: Almost half of the homes of asthmatic children contain an adult who smokes. A significant effort should be made to educate the parents and to convince them to stop smoking.

Emotions: Emotional stress and psychopathology, especially depression or a child's manipulative induction of the asthma attack, can increase the likelihood of a fatal outcome in children. Childhood is a uniquely dependent stage of life, and family stress or psychopathology may indirectly interfere with an asthmatic child's care. Compliance is an issue in adolescent asthmatics, as it is with any chronic disease of this age. The issue is best managed by beginning to deal individually with the adolescent, by always suspecting problems with drug compliance and asking about it, and by providing consistent, honest advice regarding consequences.

Pharmacotherapy

Goals of asthma therapy are multidirectional: 1) provide a bronchodilator to relieve bronchospasm, 2) protect the airways

from irritant stimuli and prevent inflammatory
gens, and 3) resolve the inflammatory process in
7-1 summarizes available information regarding
effects of each medication class based on these g

Medications may be grouped into bror
adrenergic agonists, theophylline, and antich   ─g.cs) and
nonbronchodilators (cromolyn and glucocorticoids).

Nonbronchodilators—cromolyn: International consensus guidelines
suggest that cromolyn be considered as the first line of intervention
for children manifesting frequent symptoms (those who need
β-adrenergic agonists >3 times a week). Cromolyn's primary advantage is the minimal incidence of adverse effects. Beneficial
effects relate to cromolyn's prophylactic effect for allergen- and
exercise-induced asthma. It has unique properties of blocking
early- and late-phase pulmonary responses to allergen challenge.
With chronic therapy, symptoms improve and airway hyperresponsiveness reduces.

As the severity of asthma increases, beneficial effects of
cromolyn are less obvious and the drug adds little to severe asthma.
Cromolyn is administered as a dry powder (20 mg Spinhaler), a
solution for nebulization (20 mg/2 ml solution), or a metered-dose
inhaler (MDI) (1 mg/actuation). Initial dosing should be 3 to 4
times a day with either 20 mg by nebulizer or two inhalations by
MDI. With symptom control, frequency may be decreased as
tolerated by the patient.

Table 7-1. Comparative Effects of Asthma Medications

| Medication | Bronchodilator | Protection | | Long-term Resolution[a] |
		Allergen[b]	Histamine	
Nonbronchodilator antiasthma medications				
Cromolyn	−	I, L, AR	−	+ +
Nedocromil	−	I, L, AR	−	+ + +
Glucocorticoids	−	L, AR	−	+ + +
Bronchodilators				
β-adrenergics	+ + +	I	+ + +	−
Theophylline	+ +	I, L	+	+
Anticholinergics	+	−	ND	ND

+ + +, marked effect; + +, moderate effect; +, some effect; −, no effect; ND, no data.
[a] Resolution is defined as a reduction in airway hyperresponsiveness with chronic therapy.
[b] Allergen challenge: I, immediate; LR, late phase; AR, airway hyperreactivity.

121

romil: This is another nonsteroidal antiasthma medication. Nedocromil may provide the advantage of greater potency than cromolyn and an extended mechanism of beneficial effect as well as having an additive effect with inhaled glucocorticoids. Nedocromil is available in a metered-dose aerosol formulation and a solution for nebulization (outside the U.S.) Taste pervasion remains as a major deterrent to its use in children.

Inhaled glucocorticoids: These represent the most potent anti-inflammatory agents available for the treatment of asthma. When administered prior to an allergen challenge in a sensitized patient, they block the late-phase pulmonary response and the development of airway hyperresponsiveness. Continued administration of inhaled glucocorticoid therapy is also effective in reducing the immediate pulmonary response to an allergen challenge. Inhaled glucocorticoids are also more effective than β-adrenergic agonists, theophylline, and cromolyn in reducing airway hyperresponsiveness during maintenance treatment.

Maximum dosing guidelines for inhaled glucocorticoids in children are listed in Table 7-2. More studies are needed to establish safety for doses that exceed product recommendations. Studies in adults suggest that high-dose inhaled glucocorticoids ($>1000\,\mu g$ per day) may affect skin thickness, serum osteocalcin (a protein synthesized by osteoblasts and associated with bone formation), and bone densitometry. Studies in children indicate that doses approaching $800\,\mu g$ per day may alter growth rates. Because of the risk of systemic absorption, children should be taught to use a spacer for medication administration and rinse the mouth after inhaling the dose.

Table 7-2. Maximum Recommended Adult and Pediatric Doses for Available Inhaled Glucocorticoids

Glucocorticoid	Concentrations (μg/inhalation)	Adults		Children[a]	
		inhalations/ day	mg/day	inhalations/ day	mg/day
Beclomethasone dipropionate	42	20	0.84	10	0.42
Triamcinolone acetonide	100	16	1.6	12	1.2
Flunisolide	250	8	2.0	4	1.0

[a] Pediatric doses are prescribed for children 6 to 12 years old.

Systemic glucocorticoid therapy: Oral glucocorticoids may be administered to maximize pulmonary function, reduce inflammation, and allow for maximal deposition of inhaled medications. The prednisone dose can then be tapered, supplemented, and eventually totally replaced by inhaled glucocorticoids. Starting doses consist of 2 mg/kg/day divided into two equal doses for four to seven days, depending on clinical response. If this schedule is continued beyond two weeks, a tapering schedule is recommended. In patients with very difficult asthma, the objective is to utilize the lowest oral glucocorticoid dose, if possible given on alternate days, to minimize symptoms and risk from glucocorticoid complications.

Bronchodilators

These medications are now viewed as supplementary to the nonbronchodilator antiasthma medications.

β-Adrenergic agonists: This group of medications consists of some relatively short-acting medications (epinephrine, isoproterenol) to those of moderate duration of action (albuterol, terbutaline, pirbuterol) lasting four to six hours to those with 12-hour duration. Their greatest advantage is a rapid onset of effect in the relief of acute bronchospasm via smooth muscle relaxation. These medications are the treatment of choice for acute asthma exacerbations and excellent bronchoprotective agents for pretreatment prior to exercise. β-Adrenergic agonists are administered primarily through inhalation, via either nebulized solution or metered-dose aerosol delivery. In young children, oral solutions may be useful on an intermittent basis and oral β-adrenergic agonists in the form of delayed delivery systems (Proventil-Repetabs®, Schering Corp.) may be helpful in controlling nocturnal exacerbations.

Theophylline: In the mid-1980s, theophylline was considered the drug of choice for first-line therapy in asthmatic children in the United States. Although a weak bronchodilator when compared to β-adrenergic agonists, the main advantage of theophylline is the long duration of action, 10 to 12 hours, especially useful in the management of nocturnal asthma. Theophylline has moderate bronchoprotective effects with regard to exercise and histamine challenge; it also attenuates the early- and late-phase pulmonary response to an allergen challenge. This may be related to potential anti-inflammatory properties, since it decreases microvascular leakage and macrophage activity.

Other advantages for children include its ease of administration, feasibility of once or twice daily dosing, ability to individualize dose and monitor compliance, reduction in the number of days with asthma symptoms and need for extra β-agonist treatments, improved exercise tolerance, reduced nocturnal symptoms, and reduced steroid requirement in patients with steroid-dependent asthma.

The disadvantages of theophylline therapy include a low margin of safety, multiple conditions affecting theophylline absorption and elimination, potential adverse effects related to behavior, and potential for drug interactions with readily available medications such as erythromycin. Concern has been raised regarding the possible effects of viral infections or fever on theophylline elimination. These issues, as well as others, have been addressed in several recent reviews.

Children well maintained on theophylline therapy have demonstrated signs of toxicity during the course of a fever or viral illness. Patients and parents should be cautioned regarding the possibility of altered theophylline elimination during respiratory infections, particularly with fever, and guidelines for management should be established. If fever persists for 24 hours, the physician should be contacted for further recommendations (i.e., dosage reduction or measurement of serum theophylline concentration).

Patients may require high doses of theophylline because of rapid theophylline elimination, impaired or erratic theophylline absorption, or misinterpretation of low serum theophylline concentrations during inconsistent compliance. The noncompliant patient may receive the medication on a more consistent basis during acute illnesses, possibly leading to systemic accumulation and increased serum theophylline concentration and toxicity. A ceiling on theophylline dose is recommended at 28 mg/kg/day.

For infants less than one year of age, in whom the rate of metabolism slowly increases with maturation, the initial total daily doses can be calculated from the formula

$$\text{mg/kg/day} = (0.2) \text{ (age in weeks)} + 5.0$$

For children over one year of age, the initial dose recommendation has been 16 mg/kg/day, up to a maximum of 400 mg per day. Even greater assurance of tolerance can be provided by beginning at no higher than 12 to 14 mg/kg/day (average weight for height should be used for obese patients) up to a maximum of 300 mg/

day. In children who weigh less than 45 kg the dose can be increased, if tolerated, to 16 mg/kg/day up to a maximum of 400 mg/day. If this is tolerated, the dose can be further increased to 20 mg/kg/day up to a maximum of 600 mg/day and a serum concentration measured after three days of this dose.

Parents should be instructed to discontinue theophylline if it causes adverse effects. Theophylline therapy is then resumed at a lower, previously tolerated dose. The eventual dose should be guided by a measurement of peak serum concentration. Interpretations of serum concentrations can be complicated; therefore, the "therapeutic range" should be adjusted to 8 to 15 µg/ml to allow for variability in theophylline absorption or elimination.

Anticholinergics: This group of medications apparently has limited application in the treatment of asthma. Studies in severely asthmatic patients suggest that anticholinergics provide additive effects to β-adrenergic agonists, and higher doses, administered via nebulizer, may extend the duration of effect of β-adrenergic agonists.

THE WHEEZING INFANT

Asthma in infancy presents challenges in diagnosis, management of allergic components, severity and treatment of acute attacks, and drug therapy.

Diagnosis

The diagnosis of asthma in infants is difficult since a third of all infants wheeze at least once during the first year, usually due to respiratory infections. Many children may ultimately develop asthma, but more commonly infants wheeze once or twice with viral infections and then have no further problems. The most common cause of recurrent lower respiratory cough and wheeze in infants is simply recurrent colds, especially in daycare settings. Asthma is the second most common cause, but congenital anomalies (vascular ring, tracheal esophageal fistulae, and congenital heart disease), metabolic abnormalities (cystic fibrosis), foreign body aspiration, immune deficiency syndromes, and gastroesophageal reflux must be considered.

Evaluation

Any infant with recurrent wheezing should have a careful review of systems, a chest x-ray, and a careful physical examination.

Laboratory evaluation and confirmation of an allergy history in infants are more difficult because skin tests are generally nonreactive in infants and radioallergosorbent tests (RAST) are more likely to be negative. Food allergens are clearly related to symptoms in wheezing infants with positive skin or RAST tests, and food challenges induce respiratory symptoms in at least 30% of all infants with positive tests. Sensitivity to inhalant allergens (dust mite, cat, dog) can be demonstrated occasionally in the first year but become demonstrable by age three.

Infants with asthma probably should receive prick skin tests for common food (milk, egg, wheat, soy) and inhalant allergens (dust mite, cat, dog, helminthosporium, aspergillus). Avoidance procedures are indicated for any positive tests.

Acute attacks: Infants tend to have more severe acute attacks of asthma, be more resistant to treatment, and be more vulnerable to respiratory failure. Several factors may be responsible, including greater resting resistance in small peripheral airways at this age; decreased elastic recoil, which would predispose to small airway collapse; and decreased collateral ventilation. These factors may predispose to persistent wheezing and to the characteristic picture of the "happy wheezer" (i.e., the infant who thrives and appears to ventilate adequately despite persistent audible wheezing that does not respond to bronchodilator therapy). The chest wall of the infant is more flexible and unstable, and the diaphragm contains fewer red spindles so that the strength to ventilate past the increased resistance of acute asthma and the endurance to sustain that effort are diminished.

Treatment: Response to bronchodilator therapy in infants is not striking, especially during an acute episode. Aerosolized medication usually must be given with a nebulizer. Some infants tolerate a face mask, while others allow the nebulizer outlet only to be held close to the face while sitting in the parent's lap. A great deal of support for the parent and imaginative methods for increasing acceptance by the infant are required. Solutions of glucocorticoids appropriate for nebulization are not currently available in the U.S. Therefore, steroid therapy must be given orally. A number of liquid oral steroid preparations are available, including prednisone (Pediapred®, 5 mg/teaspoonful) and prednisolone (Prelone®, 15 mg/teaspoonful), but infants often object to the taste of these preparations.

HIGH-RISK ASTHMA

It is extremely important to recognize situations predisposing to high risk for asthma mortality and to attempt to address significant problems. These children can be identified through frequent emergency-room visits, intensive-care-unit admissions, and a history of assisted ventilation. Dysfunctional families and significant socioeconomic problems also contribute to high risk, especially if associated with patient denial of illness and poor adherence to the prescribed treatment program. In these situations, the feasibility of social service and psychological assistance should be evaluated.

EXERCISE-INDUCED ASTHMA: CLINICAL MANIFESTATIONS

Exercise-induced asthma (EIA) was described as early as the seventeenth century and is a normal feature of childhood and young adult asthma. Some asthmatics develop bronchospasm if they hyperventilate, and even the deep breaths used to perform lung function tests could provoke an attack. This condition is identified as hyperventilation-induced asthma (HIA) and resembles EIA in many ways with a similar time course. Herxheimer in 1946 and Jones and his colleagues in the early sixties pioneered the scientific investigations that characterized the asthmatic attack provoked by exercise or hyperventilation. The diminution of response to further exercise after an initial attack of EIA—a refractory period—has been described. The basic mechanism of EIA, HIA, and osmotically induced asthma (OIA) is still under investigation, yet all three types of asthma are seen clinically.

Lung function changes in EIA

Changes in lung function occur within six minutes of reasonably hard exercise (Figure 7-1). During the actual period of exercise, lung function changes little or may even improve, yet toward the end of exercise, lung function begins to deteriorate in a way that can be quite marked. The major fall in lung function normally occurs five to ten minutes after stopping. Lung function normally returns spontaneously to baseline over 30 to 45 minutes. Despite similarity between EIA and the early phase of allergen-induced asthma, late-phase responses are not seen after EIA.

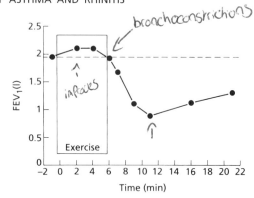

bronchoconstrictions

inflates

Figure 7-1. Typical pattern of exercise-induced asthma. Note that during exercise there is some improvement in lung function and bronchoconstriction occurs only after stopping. SOURCE: Godfrey S. Exercise-induced asthma. In: Bierman CW, Pearlman DS, eds. Allergic diseases from infancy to adulthood. Philadelphia: WB Saunders, 1988:597–606.

EIA, bronchial hyperreactivity, and atopy

EIA is generally believed to be a manifestation of the increased airway reactivity characteristic of asthma and demonstrable by other means. This hyperreactivity is an order of magnitude greater in asthma compared with normal subjects or patients with other lung diseases. Mellis et al studied 50 asthmatic children and compared their responses to exercise and to histamine. They found a correlation between the responses to the two challenges, although the incidence of a positive response was greater with histamine (90%) than with exercise (74%). A similar conclusion was reached in another study, in which 95% of asthmatics responded to a methacholine challenge, 71% to ultrasonic fog, and 57% to cold-air hyperventilation. Increased bronchial reactivity has been noted in patients other than asthmatics, such as those with hay fever, formerly wheezy infants, relatives of asthmatic children, and wheezy infants and children with cystic fibrosis. In all these groups the lability consists mainly of increased bronchodilatation during exercise and a small increase in postexercise bronchoconstriction, far less than that seen in asthma.

The incidence of EIA in asthmatics and the reproducibility of tests of EIA are greatly influenced by the nature of the exercise test and the conditions under which the exercise is performed. With random testing of asthmatics of average severity, it appears that about 70 to 90% will develop a fall in FEV_1 that is outside the normal range.

Pharmacological modification of EIA

EIA can be inhibited by the prior administration of sympathomimetic agents but not by steroids or antihistamines. The value of theophylline derivatives and atropine was less certain. Cromolyn sodium also blocked EIA.

While sympathomimetic agents are very potent inhibitors of EIA, there is some doubt as to the relative efficacy of oral versus inhaled preparations, even though bronchodilatation occurs after administration by either route. Anderson et al found oral salbutamol to be ineffective compared with the inhaled drug, but Francis et al found both forms to be equally effective.

Recently, interest in other agents showed promising results with nifedipine. Ketotifen, an antihistaminic compound, totally failed to inhibit EIA in carefully controlled studies, yet terfenadine did show blocking of EIA and OIA but not of HIA. More exciting, the diuretic furosemide also can block both EIA and OIA when given by inhalation.

A refractory period has been demonstrated after both EIA and HIA. The refractory period following EIA can be eliminated by treatment with indomethacin, while the drug has no effect on the refractory period following HIA.

For practical purposes, a patient with EIA should be given either a selective β_2-sympathomimetic or cromolyn sodium immediately before exercise by inhalation. In absolute terms the sympathomimetic is more effective and its duration is longer, but it requires a perfect inhalation technique. Protection falls to about 50% of initial protection in about 4 to 5 hours with salbutamol and in 1.5 to 2 hours with cromolyn. There is no logical reason to use theophylline, either short- or long-acting, for the sole purpose of inhibiting EIA.

SELECTED REFERENCES

American Academy of Allergy and Immunology Study Group. Comparison of aerosol beclomethasone and oral theophylline as primary treatment of chronic asthma: III, adverse effects. J Allergy Clin Immunol 1991;87:202 (abs).

Anderson SD. Is there a unifying hypothesis for exercise induced asthma? J Allergy Clin Immunol 1984;73:660–665.

Anderson SD, Seale JP, Rozea P, et al. Inhaled and oral salbutamol in exercise induced asthma. Am Rev Respir Dis 1976;114: 493–500.

Bar-Yishay E, Godfrey S. Exercise induced asthma. In: Weiss EB, Segal MS, and Stein M. Bronchial asthma: mechanisms and therapeutics. 3rd ed. Boston: Little Brown & Co., 1993, ch. 47.

Blair J. Natural history of childhood asthma: 20 year follow-up. Arch Dis Child 1977;52:613–619.

Boulet L-P, Legris C, Turcotte H, Hebert J. Prevalence and characteristics of late asthmatic responses to exercise. J Allergy Clin Immunol 1987;80:655–662.

Committee on Drugs, American Academy of Pediatrics. Precautions concerning the use of theophylline. Pediatrics 1992;89: 781–783.

Davies SE. The effect of disodium cromoglycate on exercise induced asthma. Br Med J 1968;3:593–594.

Evans R III, Mullally DI, Wilson RW, et al. National trends in morbidity and mortality of asthma in the US: prevalence, hospitalization rate and death from asthma over two decades (1965–1984). Chest 1987;91:65s–74s.

Finnerty JP, Wilmot C, Holgate ST. Inhibition of hypertonic saline induced bronchoconstriction by terfenadine and flurbiprafen. Am Rev Respir Dis 1989;140:593–597.

Floyer J, Sir. A treatise of the asthma. London: R. Wilkin and W. Innis, 1698.

Francis PW, Krastins IR, Levison H. Oral and inhaled salbutamol in the prevention of exercise induced bronchospasm. Pediatrics 1980;66:103–108.

Galdes-Sebaldt M, McLaughlin FJ, Levison H. Comparison of cold air, ultrasonic mist, and methacholine inhalations as tests of bronchial reactivity in normal and asthmatic children. J Pediatr 1985;107:526–530.

Gergen PJ, Mullally DI, Evans R. National survey of prevalence of asthma among children in the United States (1976–1980). Pediatrics 1988;81:1–7.

Hendeles L, Weinberger M, Szefler S, Ellis E. Safety and efficacy of theophylline in children with asthma? J Pediatr 1992;89: 177–183.

Herxheimer H. Hyperventilation asthma. Lancet 1946;1:83–87.

Hudgel DW, Langston L Jr, Selner JC, McIntosh K. Viral and bacterial infections in adults with chronic asthma. Am Rev Resp Dis 1979;120:393–397.

International Consensus Report on Diagnosis and Treatment of Asthma. National Heart, Lung and Blood Institute, National Institutes of Health, Publication No. 92-3091, Bethesda, Maryland, March 1992.

Joad JP, Ahrens RC, Lindgren SD, Weinberger MM. Relative efficacy of maintenance therapy with theophylline, inhaled albuterol, and the combination for chronic asthma. J Allergy Clin Immunol 1987;79:78–85.

Jones RS, Wharton MJ, Buston MH. The place of physical exercise and bronchodilator drugs in the assessment of the asthmatic child. Arch Dis Child 1963;38:539–545.

Kattan M, Keens TG, Lapierre J-G, et al. Pulmonary function abnormalities in symptom-free children after bronchiolitis. Pediatrics 1977;59:683–688.

Kennedy JD, Hasham F, Clay MJD, Jones RS. Comparision of actions of disodium cromoglycate and ketotifen on exercise induced bronchoconstriction in childhood asthma. Br Med J 1980;281:1458.

Kjellman NM, Croner S. Cord blood IgE determination for allergy prediction—a follow-up study of seven (7) years of age and 1,651 children. Ann Allergy 1984;53:167–171.

McFadden ER. Hypothesis: exercise-induced asthma as a vascular phenomenon. Lancet 1990;335:880–883.

Mellis CM, Kattan M, Keens TG, Levison H. Comparative study of histamine and exercise challenges in asthmatic children. Am Rev Respir Dis 1978;117:911–915.

Mullally DI, Howard WA, Hubbard TJ. Increased hospitalizations for asthma among children in the Washington DC area during 1961–1981. Ann Allergy 1984;53:15–19.

Pauwels R, Van Renterghem D, Van der Straeten M, et al. The effect of theophylline and enprofylline on allergen-induced bronchoconstriction. J Allergy Clin Immunol 1985;76:583–590.

Pouw EM, Prummel MF, Oosting H, Roos CM, Endert E. Beclomethasone inhalation decreases serum osteocalcin concentrations. Br Med J 1991;302:627–628.

Rebuck AS, Keston S, Boulet L, et al. A 3-month evaluation of nedocromil sodium in asthma: a randomized, double-blind, placebo-controlled trial of nedocromil sodium conducted by a

Canadian multicenter study group. J Allergy Clin Immunol 1990;85:612–617.

Szefler SJ. Alternative therapy in asthma: rationale and guidelines for applications. In: Middleton E Jr, Reed CE, Ellis EF, et al., eds. Update #11 for allergy: principles and practice. 3rd ed. St Louis: CV Mosby, 1991:1–14.

Szefler SJ. Anti-inflammatory drugs in the treatment of allergic disease. Med Clin North Am 1992;6:953–975.

Szefler SJ. Glucocorticoid therapy for asthma: clinical pharmacology. J Allergy Clin Immunol 1991;88:147–165.

Vichyanond P, Sladek WA, Sur S, et al. Efficacy of atropine methylnitrate alone and in combination with albuterol in children with asthma. Chest 1990;98:637–642.

Williams J, McNichol KN. Prevalence and natural history in relationship of wheezing bronchitis and asthma in children: an epidemiologic study. Br Med J 1969;3:321–325.

Zeiger RS. Development and prevention of allergic disease in childhood. In: Middleton EF Jr, Reed CE, Ellis EF, et al., eds. Allergy: principles and practice. 2nd ed. St Louis: CV Mosby Co., 1988:930–968.

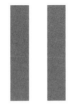

Special Problems

Management of Exacerbation of Asthma in Adults

8

INTRODUCTION

Exacerbations of asthma range from a gradual deterioration with increasing symptoms to a precipitous severe attack in which death may be imminent. Although the management of these different situations may vary, the basic approach is similar: to assess the severity of the attack; to institute appropriate therapy; to assess the response to treatment, thereby identifying patients requiring more intensive therapy; and to undertake follow-up to ensure that complete recovery is achieved and the risk of further exacerbations is reduced.

Mortality surveys have consistently found that failure by the patient to assess and appreciate the severity of his or her asthma, resulting in a delay in instituting appropriate therapy, is a major contributory factor to a fatal outcome. As a result, most deaths from asthma occur before the patient has received medical attention. If a significant impact is to be made on morbidity and mortality from severe asthma, attention must be focused on the ways in which asthmatic patients can successfully recognize and self-manage severe exacerbations of their disease.

PATIENT SELF-MANAGEMENT OF WORSENING ASTHMA

A life-threatening attack requiring hospital admission usually develops after some considerable period of instability and worsening control. During this period, opportunities exist for the asthmatic patient to recognize deteriorating asthma and institute appropriate treatment, thereby reducing the probability of developing a life-threatening attack.

Assessment of severity

The most common way in which a patient attempts to determine the severity of his or her asthma is by the perception of symptoms such as breathlessness, wheeze, and chest tightness. However, this method may be inadequate, as impairment in airway caliber is not always readily perceived by patients. A significant number of chronic adult asthmatics have minimal symptoms despite marked airflow obstruction (as measured by reduction in the forced expiratory flow in one second, FEV_1, from predicted values). Patients with the most severe asthma have the worst perception of the degree of airflow obstruction, suggesting that adaptation over time may be in part responsible for this phenomenon. It also indicates that patients who are at greatest risk of a severe attack of asthma are those most likely to underestimate the severity of such an attack, and provides a reason for the finding that delay in seeking emergency medical assistance commonly contributes to a fatal outcome. Similar difficulty exists in the clinical situation of recovery from a severe attack of asthma, in which most asthmatic patients become symptom-free despite the mean FEV_1 reaching only 50% of the predicted normal. Even patients experiencing major disability with severe symptoms may not recognize their importance. One study found that about one-fifth of patients tested with a hypothetical asthma attack delayed seeking medical help despite having severe symptoms.

It is now recognized that, in addition to changes in symptoms, objective measurements of airflow obstruction are necessary if asthmatic patients (and their physicians) are to assess more accurately the severity of their deteriorating asthma. While measurement of FEV_1 is recognized as a "gold standard," measurement of the peak expiratory flow rate (PEFR) is an acceptable alternative which offers the advantage of being cheaper, more portable, and simpler to use. With instruction, the PEFR is a highly repeatable measurement, and there is a good correlation between it and the FEV_1. Predicted normal values have been calculated based on age, sex, and height. Measurements of PEFR are most easily interpreted when expressed as a percentage of the predicted normal value or of the previous best obtainable value on optimal treatment.

However, it is not sufficient for patients to measure changes in PEFR; they need a system whereby they can interpret the changes, in order to recognize the severity of their asthma and to undertake the appropriate therapeutic responses. For this purpose, it is necessary for the patient to have a written self-management plan.

Self-management plans

Self-management plans focus on the early recognition of unstable or deteriorating asthma through interpretation of peak flow recordings and symptoms. Through the use of written treatment guidelines, patients are able to determine when adjustments to therapy are required and when it is necessary to call for appropriate medical assistance. Most self-management plans include three or four broad stages based on the decrease in peak flow from the patient's previous best recordings and/or the development of worsening symptoms and an increasing requirement for inhaled β-agonist therapy. For each stage of deterioration, clear instructions are written as to what self-management steps the patient should take and when to seek medical help. The therapeutic intervention is tailored to the individual patient and his or her requirements.

Several self-management plans have been recommended, varying with respect to the amount of detail they provide, the specific drug treatment recommended at each stage, and the level of decrease in peak flow or severity of symptoms chosen for the various therapeutic responses recommended. The difficulty with the application of these self-management plans is that few have been formally tested. Furthermore, the requirements of individual asthmatic patients may vary considerably, meaning that no single plan is likely to be suitable for every patient. As a result of these difficulties, features such as the precise level (or range of levels) of peak flow (whether pre- or post-bronchodilator) at which patients are advised to modify therapy or seek medical assistance have not been clearly established. It is with these limitations in mind that the various self-management plans should be viewed; a home self-management plan based on the International Consensus Report guidelines is found in Figure 8-1.

The patient can recognize the first stage of stable asthma by a pre-bronchodilator peak flow of above 80% of best, few symptoms, and the infrequent need for use of a bronchodilator aerosol. At this level, most patients can be maintained on twice daily inhaled anti-inflammatory therapy together with a β-agonist inhaler for use as required to relieve symptoms. For most patients, the anti-

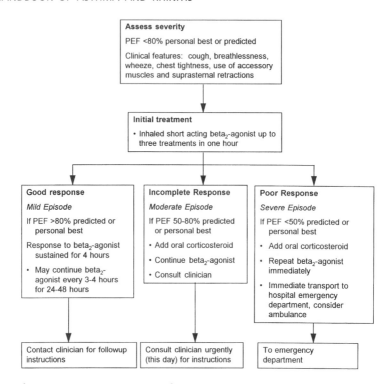

Figure 8-1. Management of Exacerbation of Asthma: Home Treatment. SOURCE: International Consensus Report on Diagnosis and Treatment of Asthma. National Heart, Lung and Blood Institute, National Institute of Health, Bethesda, MD, March 1992 [Clin Exp Allergy 1992; 22(suppl 1)].

inflammatory therapy will be inhaled. Anti-inflammatory therapy emphasizes to the patient the importance of this form of therapy and encourages compliance; it also serves to overcome the reduced drug deposition that occurs in this clinical situation. The recommended way to double the dose is increasing the frequency of administration from twice daily to four times daily, a regimen which has been shown to result in greater efficacy. The dose is reduced to its previous level after control is achieved. At this stage, and all other stages, inhaled bronchodilator therapy is recommended as required by the patient to relieve symptoms but should not be dosed on a regular, scheduled regimen.

If the patient frequently has to double the dose of inhaled anti-inflammatory medication, in accordance with the second stage, then this higher dose becomes the regular daily dose taken by the patient. In this way the self-management plan can be used to determine the dose of regular anti-inflammatory therapy required by the patient to ensure long-term control. Similarly, the self-management plan can be used by the patients to reduce treatment following a prolonged period of good control. Thus, if the patient has remained in the first stage for a number of months, with few symptoms and normal lung function, he or she can be instructed to reduce (initially halve) the dose of the inhaled anti-inflammatory therapy, while continuing to monitor the asthma in case a deterioration occurs.

This method of varying the dose of inhaled anti-inflammatory medication over longer periods of time is consistent with the recommendations for the long-term management of chronic persistent asthma in adults, in which a stepwise approach to asthma therapy based on the classification of the severity of the asthma is proposed. Its incorporation into a patient self-management plan represents one way in which the recommendations for acute severe and chronic persistent asthma can be brought together within the framework of one system.

A poor response to the increased use of inhaled β-agonist medication together with a further fall in pre-bronchodilator peak flow to below about 40 to 60% of the best level is an indicator of a severe attack. At this third stage, the patient is instructed to start oral corticosteroids and contact the physician. High doses of an orally administered corticosteroid, begun early in this way, can prevent a protracted or progressive course and reduce the requirement for emergency care or hospitalization. It is not possible to determine, at this stage, the likely rate of recovery from the attack, and as a result, how long the patient will need to continue oral corticosteroid therapy. For this reason, fixed-dose regimens should be avoided, although three doses of 30 to 60 mg of prednisone per day are commonly used. Instead, the patient is encouraged to continue taking a high dose of oral corticosteroids until the peak flow returns to normal values; according to individual preference, either the patient would then take half the dose for the same number of days before stopping, or the dose could be tapered more gradually over this period. Thus, the aim of this regimen is to start oral corticosteroids in sufficient dosage early in an attack and to use the subsequent therapeutic response to determine the duration of treatment.

As with the previous stage, assessment of the response to bronchodilator treatment is used to determine the need for emergency medical management. A level of peak flow <40% of best and a minimal response to frequent inhaled β-agonist medication represent the requirement for emergency medical help (Stage 4). There is a good rationale for these guidelines, as falls in peak flow of >50% have been shown to precede sudden death, and the requirement for very high doses of inhaled β-agonist therapy has also been shown to be a good marker for risk of a fatal or near-fatal attack of asthma.

For the successful implementation of such a self-management plan based on PEFR recordings, it is necessary for the personal best PEFR value to be determined for each patient. If the patient's best PEFRs are significantly below the predicted normal values, then more aggressive therapy, such as a two-week course of oral corticosteroids, may be required to determine if a higher personal best value is achievable. The highest PEFR measurement consistently achieved after such a period of maximum therapy is then taken as the patient's best value, against which subsequent measurements are evaluated.

PRECIPITOUS ASTHMA

Most patients who develop severe asthma have had progressively worsening asthma over a period of days or weeks. Some patients, however, have recurrent precipitous attacks in which they develop severe, life-threatening asthma within minutes or hours, with little instability of asthma in the preceding days. The educated use of a self-management plan is particularly important with these patients, with the plan modified so that each stage is set at a higher level; thus, emergency treatment can be initiated earlier in the attack. Some additional resources such as the availability of oxygen in the patient's home and a nebulizer to administer high doses of a β-agonist are also recommended. If resources are not available to provide a nebulizer, multiple doses of a β-agonist via a spacer is an acceptable alternative. The provision of a syringe preloaded with epinephrine for subcutaneous injection and other resuscitation equipment should be considered. Patients need to recognize that these therapeutic measures are to be undertaken while medical attention is urgently sought and are not a substitute for medical assessment and treatment.

The facility for self-referral and admission to the hospital should exist, and this may require prior arrangement with the ambulance service. The advantages of such a service, which gives immediate admission without the need for medical referral to known high-risk patients with a previous life-threatening attack, have been shown. In addition to the patients, their relatives and friends should be familiar with the plan for management, including the administration of the drugs.

Medical assessment and treatment

The approach to the management of a patient with severe asthma is similar regardless of the medical setting. The priorities are to assess the severity through objective methods, identify the high-risk patients, institute appropriate therapy, and assess the response to treatment to determine those in need of hospital admission and those requiring more intensive therapy (Figure 8-2).

Assessment of severity

When attending a patient with an exacerbation of asthma, the physician should undertake a brief history and physical examination, together with a functional assessment of the severity of the attack, as therapy is started (Table 8-1). The purpose of the initial brief history is to identify characteristics of the patient's past history that indicate a high-risk patient, as well as those features which suggest that there is a potentially life-threatening attack. A brief cardiopulmonary examination should also be performed, with emphasis on findings relevant to assessing the severity of the attack and to identifying complications or alternative diagnoses such as heart failure.

Objective measurement of the degree of airflow obstruction before and after bronchodilator therapy by use of PEFR or FEV_1 is the most important method of assessing the severity of an attack of asthma in this situation. Such measurements are more reliable than other clinical or laboratory parameters as indicators of the degree of obstruction and the likely requirement for more intensive therapy. Whereas a peak flow meter may be more suitable for use in a patient's home, or an office setting or for serial measurements in the hospital, a spirometer with measurement of FEV_1 offers a better alternative for hospital emergency department use. Depending on the severity of the attack, measurement of arterial blood gases and chest radiography may be necessary in severe cases.

Initial Assessment

History (hx) physical examination (auscultation, use of accessory muscles, heart rate, respiratory rate, PEF or FEV_1, oxygen saturation, arterial blood gas of patient in extremis, and other tests as indicated

Initial Treatment

Inhaled short acting beta$_2$-agonist, usually by nebulization, one dose every 20min for 1 hour

Oxygen to achieve O_2 saturation ≥90% (95% children)

Systemic corticosteroids if no immediate response or if patient recently took oral steroid, or if episode is severe

Sedation is contraindicated in the treatment of exacerbations

Repeat Assessment

PE, PEF, O_2 saturation, other tests as needed

Severe Episode

PEF <50% predicted / personal best

Physical exam: severe symptoms at rest, chest retraction

Hx: high risk patient

No improvement after initial treatment

inhaled beta$_2$-agonist, hourly or continuous ± inhaled anticholinergic

Oxygen

Systemic corticosteroid

Consider subcutaneous, intramuscular, or intravenous beta$_2$-agonist

Moderate Episode

PEF 50–70% predicted / personal best

Physical exam: moderate symptoms, accessory muscle use

Inhaled beta$_2$-agonist every 60 minutes

Consider corticosteroids

Continue treatment 1–3 hours, provided there is improvement

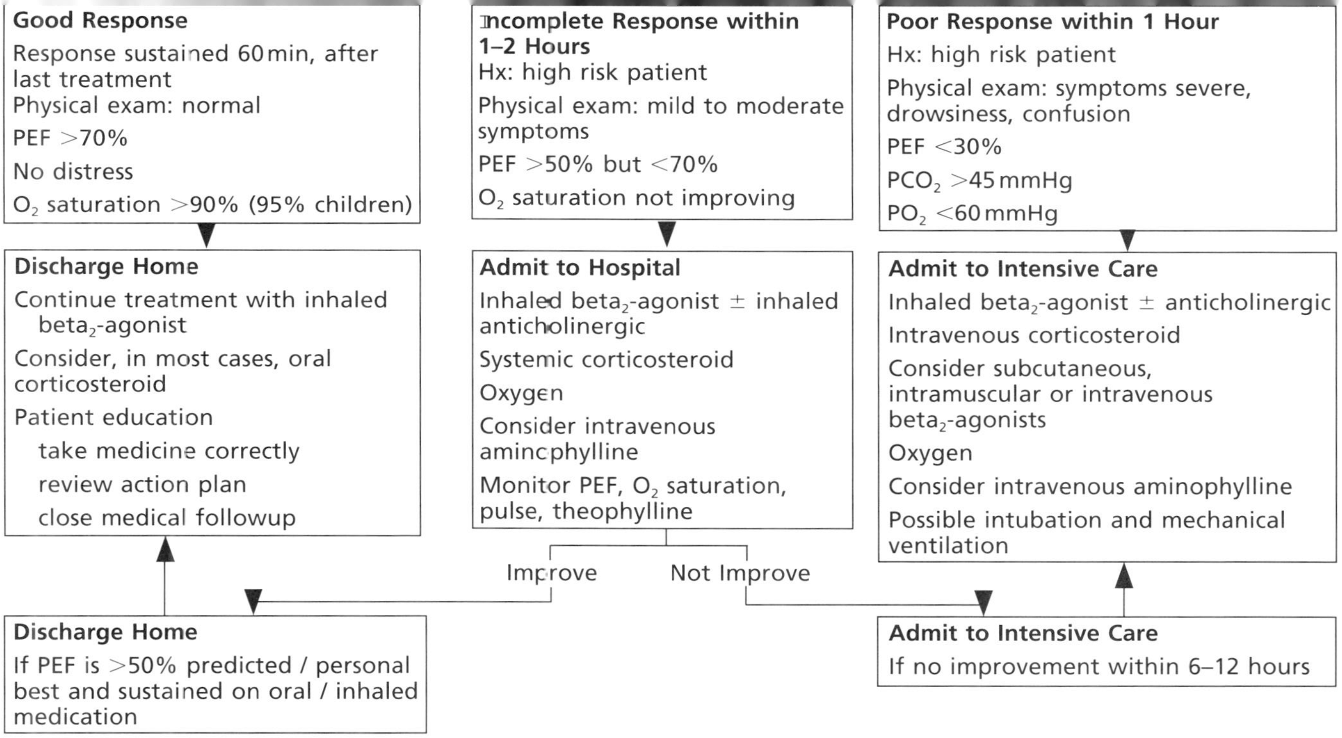

Good Response

Response sustained 60 min, after last treatment

Physical exam: normal

PEF >70%

No distress

O$_2$ saturation >90% (95% children)

Incomplete Response within 1–2 Hours

Hx: high risk patient

Physical exam: mild to moderate symptoms

PEF >50% but <70%

O$_2$ saturation not improving

Poor Response within 1 Hour

Hx: high risk patient

Physical exam: symptoms severe, drowsiness, confusion

PEF <30%

PCO$_2$ >45 mmHg

PO$_2$ <60 mmHg

Discharge Home

Continue treatment with inhaled beta$_2$-agonist

Consider, in most cases, oral corticosteroid

Patient education

take medicine correctly

review action plan

close medical followup

Admit to Hospital

Inhaled beta$_2$-agonist ± inhaled anticholinergic

Systemic corticosteroid

Oxygen

Consider intravenous aminophylline

Monitor PEF, O$_2$ saturation, pulse, theophylline

Admit to Intensive Care

Inhaled beta$_2$-agonist ± anticholinergic

Intravenous corticosteroid

Consider subcutaneous, intramuscular or intravenous beta$_2$-agonists

Oxygen

Consider intravenous aminophylline

Possible intubation and mechanical ventilation

Improve   Not Improve

Discharge Home

If PEF is >50% predicted / personal best and sustained on oral / inhaled medication

Admit to Intensive Care

If no improvement within 6–12 hours

Figure 8-2. **Management of Exacerbation of Asthma: Hospital-Based Care.** SOURCE: **International Consensus Report on Diagnosis and Treatment of Asthma. National Heart, Lung and Blood Institute, National Institute of Health, Bethesda, MD, 1992 [Clin Exp Allergy 1992; 22(suppl 1)].**

143

Table 8-1. Severity of Asthma Exacerbations[a]

Signs	Mild	Moderate	Severe	Respiratory arrest imminent
Breathlessness	Walking	Talking (Infant—softer shorter cry; difficulty feeding)	At rest (Infant—stops feeding)	
Position	Can lie down	Prefers sitting	Hunched forward	
Talks in	Sentences	Phrases	Words	
Alertness	May be agitated	Usually agitated	Usually agitated	Drowsy or confused
Respiratory rate	Increased	Increased	Often >30/min	

Guide to rates of breathing associated with respiratory distress in awake children:

Age	Normal rate
<2 months	<60/min
2–12 months	<50/min
1–5 years	<40/min
6–8 years	<30/min

Signs	Mild	Moderate	Severe	Respiratory arrest imminent
Accessory muscles and suprasternal retractions	Usually not	Usually	Usually	Paradoxical thoracoabdominal movement
Wheeze	Moderate, often only end expiratory	Loud	Usually loud	Absence of wheeze
Pulse/min	<100	100–120	>120	Bradycardia

Guide to limits of normal pulse rate in children:

	Age	Normal rate
Infants	2–12 months	<160/min
Preschool	1–2 years	<120/min
School age	2–8 years	<110/min

Pulse paradoxus	Absent <10 mmHg	May be present 10–25 mmHg	Often present >25 mmHg (adult) 20–40 mmHg (child)	Absence suggests respiratory muscle fatigue
PEF after initial bronchodilator % predicted or % personal best	Over 70–80%	Approx. 50–70%	<50% predicted or personal best (<100 L/min adults) or response lasts <2 hrs	
PaO_2 (on air)[b]	Normal Test not usually necessary	>60 mmHg	<60 mmHg Possible cyanosis	
and/or $PaCO_2$[b]	<45 mmHg	<45 mmHg	>45 mmHg: Possible respiratory failure (see text)	
SaO_2% (on air)[b]	>95%	91–95%	<90%	
	Hypercapnia (hypoventilation) develops more readily in young children than in adults and adolescents.			

[a]The presence of several parameters, but not necessarily all, indicates the general classification of the exacerbation.
[b]Kilopascals are also used internationally; conversion would be appropriate in this regard.
SOURCE: International Consensus Report on Diagnosis and Treatment of Asthma. National Heart, Lung and Blood Institute, National Institutes of Health, Bethesda, MD, 1992 [Clin Exp Allergy 1992; 22(suppl 1)].

Identification of patients requiring hospital admission

Assessment of the PEFR or FEV_1 before and after initial nebulized bronchodilator therapy is probably the best method for determining the requirement for hospital admission. This method can be used as the basis for decisions regarding management, an approach which has led to the development of flow charts for use in emergency settings.

It is recommended that those patients with any life-threatening features on initial presentation, or a FEV_1 or PEFR, of less than 50% of their best result (or absolute values of 1.5 L and 200 L/min, respectively), 15 to 30 minutes after nebulization, require emergency referral for admission to the hospital, or admission if seen in an emergency department.

The difficulty arises when the patient shows an incomplete response to initial nebulized bronchodilator therapy. In this situation, when the PEFR or FEV_1 remains between 50 and 70% of predicted best value, the use of additional features of the history and examination is helpful. Regarding the history, a lower threshold for admission is appropriate in patients who have had a recent hospital admission or a previous life-threatening attack, both markers of high-risk patients. A decision to admit may also be made in patients seen in the evening rather than earlier in the day, those with prolonged symptoms and multiple medication use before the visit, and those with poor access to medical care or where there is concern over the social circumstances or the ability of relatives to respond appropriately. The findings on clinical examination are also helpful in identifying life-threatening features and predicting the need for hospital admission, as discussed below. In adults with severe asthma, a chest radiograph is probably unnecessary unless the patient is unresponsive to treatment and is being admitted.

If the patient has made a good response, with a PEFR or FEV_1 >70% of the predicted value, and has no features to suggest a potentially life-threatening attack, then the patient need not be admitted to the hospital, although further medical follow-up and education will be required.

Identification of patients with potentially life-threatening asthma

There are a number of features of clinical examination or functional assessment that have been recognized as important markers of a potentially life-threatening attack (see Table 8-1).

CLINICAL EXAMINATION

Although the signs elicited by clinical examination are simple to elicit, it is difficult to be certain exactly what degree or level should be used to indicate a potentially life-threatening attack. One approach is to assess the degree of breathlessness, in particular whether the patient is unable to complete sentences in one breath or is too breathless to speak. Alternatively, assessment of the limitation of activity, such as whether the patient is totally confined to a chair or bed, is helpful. Classifications of the severity of asthma based entirely on these observations have been developed and are useful in identifying those with life-threatening asthma. The presence of a pulse rate >110 per minute is a good marker of a patient at risk of an adverse outcome. The absence of this degree of tachycardia does not exclude the possibility of a life-threatening attack, as some patients develop bradycardia as a premorbid event. Furthermore, tachycardia should not be ignored on the grounds that it might be due to bronchodilator medication. A corresponding level for the respiratory rate is about 25 breaths per minute. The presence of an inspiratory fall in blood pressure of >10 to 15 mmHg is another feature of severe attack. In one study, arterial paradox of >10 mmHg was never present if the FEV_1 was <20%. Others, however, have observed a poor correlation between paradox and asthma severity, which in part relates to the difficulty in undertaking the measurement in a critically ill patient.

Functional measurements

Although the FEV_1 and PEFR are important measurements of the severity of asthma, as with the clinical signs, it is uncertain exactly how the values should be interpreted. Values of <30 to 40% of predicted or best known values have been recommended as the level for recognition of a potentially life-threatening attack. If the patient's previous best values are not known, then an estimate for PEFR of about 150 to 200 L/min or FEV_1 of 1.0 to 1.5 L may be used. The objective response to a nebulized bronchodilator is also helpful; a failure of the PEFR or FEV_1 to improve by more than one third after initial treatment is a poor prognostic sign. In a study of severe asthma, patients with an initial FEV_1 of <30% who did not improve to at least 40% of the predicted value at the end of 60 minutes of intensive bronchodilator treatment were those who ultimately required prolonged emergency room therapy and/or hospital admission.

It is also recommended that arterial blood-gas tension be always measured in patients whose asthma exhibits features of a life-threatening attack. As an attack becomes more severe, the arterial carbon dioxide tension ($PaCO_2$) falls initially, due to compensatory hyperventilation, then rises back to within and then above the normal range. Thus, in a breathless asthmatic patient, a normal or high $PaCO_2$ is a marker of a life-threatening attack. In contrast, the PaO_2 falls steadily with worsening asthma, although the administration of a high-flow oxygen treatment makes interpretation more difficult.

Overall assessment

Due to the limitations of single features of an examination or objective measurements, an approach is recommended whereby all the features are interpreted together and their response to bronchodilator therapy determined. Whereas the presence of any one of the above-mentioned features is sufficient to consider the exacerbation to be potentially life-threatening, the presence of most of the features deserves special attention and awareness of the likely need for intensive care and assisted ventilation.

Identification of patients at risk of imminent death

There are a number of features in a severe attack of asthma that indicate that the patient is at risk of imminent death (see Table 8-1). These include an impaired level of consciousness with drowsiness and confusion, cyanosis, bradycardia, and the presence of a silent chest on auscultation. This latter sign indicates airways narrowing of sufficient magnitude to prevent sufficient airflow to generate a wheeze as well as failing ventilatory muscle function with decreased respiratory effort due to patient exhaustion. Although all of these features are serious prognostic signs, their absence is not necessarily reassuring since some patients may have a cardiorespiratory arrest without previously showing these features.

The measurement of arterial blood-gas tensions and PEFR or FEV_1 are particularly helpful in recognizing the patient at imminent risk of death. Hypercapnia, with a $PaCO_2$ of >45 mmHg, or persisting PaO_2 of <60 mmHg despite receiving high-flow oxygen, indicates a life-threatening attack requiring intensive monitoring and treatment. These values are usually associated with falls in FEV_1 or PEFR to less than 20% of predicted values, although considerable variability exists in this relationship.

Immediate treatment

Oxygen: Profound hypoxia may be present in patients with severe asthma, and so treatment should be started immediately with oxygen. Retention of CO_2 is not aggravated by treatment with oxygen in patients with severe asthma, since hypercapnia in this situation reflects the severity of airflow obstruction and muscle fatigue rather than decreased CO_2 drive, which may be the case in patients with chronic respiratory failure. Thus, masks delivering 24% or 28% oxygen are inappropriate; instead, the highest concentration of oxygen available should be delivered to the patient.

Inhaled bronchodilator drugs: In conjunction with oxygen therapy, high doses of an inhaled β-agonist drug should be administered to the patient (Table 8-2). Although nebulization is the preferred route, multiple actuations of a metered-dose inhaler into a spacer device may lead to equivalent bronchodilation. Irrespective of whether these drugs are administered in the general-practice setting, during transport by ambulance, or in the hospital, the β-agonist medication should be nebulized with oxygen. Nebulized albuterol or terbutaline should be given in the dose of 2.5 to 5 mg; fenoterol and isoprenaline should be avoided because of concerns relating to their adverse effects.

The importance of administering β-agonists with oxygen is highlighted by studies which have shown that β-agonist therapy may worsen hypoxia when administered in a severe attack of asthma and, conversely, that the presence of hypoxia and hypercapnia may influence the cardiovascular response to high doses of β-agonist drugs. Patients can tolerate very high doses of β-agonists in the hospital *when receiving oxygen therapy*, whereas the overuse of high-dose preparations of β-agonist drugs in the clinical situation of severe asthma in the community is more likely to lead to a fatal outcome.

Systemic corticosteroids: High-dose systemic corticosteroid therapy should be started immediately in a severe attack of asthma, following the administration of oxygen and nebulized β-agonists (see Table 8-2). Although it is uncertain whether there are significant advantages to intravenous compared with oral administration in the treatment of severe asthma, in patients who have a potentially life-threatening attack, it is recommended that steroids be administered

Table 8-2. Doses and Frequencies of Medications for an Acute Exacerbation of Asthma

Medication	Dose and frequency
β-agonists	
Inhaled	Nebulized:
Albuterol	2.5 mg in 3 mL of normal saline every 0.5–2.0 hr
Terbutaline	2.5 mg in 3 mL of normal saline every 0.5–2.0 hr
Metaproterenol	15 mg in 3 mL normal saline every 0.5–2.0 hr
Albuterol, terbutaline, metaproterenol, pirbuterol	Metered-dose inhaler: 2–4 puffs with spacer every 0.5–2.0 hr
Parenteral	
Epinephrine	0.3 mg subcutaneously every 0.5–4 hr up to 3–4 doses
Terbutaline	0.25 mg subcutaneously every 0.5 hr for up to 2 doses
Corticosteroids	
Systemic	
Methylprednisolone	60–80 mg intravenously every 6–8 hr
Hydrocortisone	2.0 mg/kg intravenously every 4 hr
Methylxanthines	
Aminophylline	5–6 mg/kg over 30 minutes loading dose, then 0.4–0.9 mg/kg/hr. Check serum level within 6 hr of loading dose. Do not give loading dose if patient is on oral theophylline. Check for drug interactions and disease states that alter clearance.

parenterally. Recommended regimens include hydrocortisone (2 to 3 mg/kg IV bolus stat and then either 0.5 mg/kg/hr as continuous infusion or 2 to 3 mg/kg IV bolus repeated every four to six hours); alternatively, methylprednisolone (60 to 80 mg) may be given as an IV bolus every six to eight hours—or 125 mg stat followed by oral treatment.

With improvement in the patient's condition, or in less severe cases, prednisone (or prednisolone) may be given orally. Oral prednisone (or prednisolone) is rapidly absorbed, and peak plasma levels are achieved within 15 minutes of oral administration. A reduction in the degree of airflow obstruction and increased adrenergic responsiveness have been demonstrated within one to three hours and reach a maximum five to nine hours after the administration of a single dose of corticosteroid. There is a dose–response relationship for oral steroids, with the maximum beneficial effect achieved at 0.6 mg/kg/day; there appears to be no greater benefit with the administration of higher doses.

Intravenous bronchodilators: If potentially life-threatening features are present, intravenous bronchodilators may also be given as a supplement to nebulized bronchodilator therapy, although there is little evidence that this results in a greater degree of bronchodilation than nebulized bronchodilator therapy alone, and the choice of agent remains controversial. Most studies have shown that intravenous administration of β-agonists offers no advantage over inhalation and that the combination of intravenous aminophylline with inhaled β-agonists does not result in greater bronchodilation than β-agonists alone, while leading to greater side effects. However, some studies have observed a small therapeutic benefit from the addition of either intravenous aminophylline (see Table 8-2) or intravenous β-agonists to nebulized β-agonist therapy.

Intravenous aminophylline is given in the dose of 5 to 6 mg/kg over 30 minutes, then infused in the dose range of 0.4 to 0.9 mg/kg per hour. A loading dose should not be given to patients who are already receiving oral theophylline treatment. The maintenance infusion rate is altered according to plasma theophylline levels, which should be measured within 24 hours. For the continuous infusion, lower doses may be required in patients with liver disease or cardiac failure and those taking cimetidine, ciprofloxacin, or erythromycin, whereas higher doses may be required in smokers.

Albuterol or terbutaline is administered in an intravenous dose of 200 μg over 10 minutes, followed by an infusion of 0.1 to 0.2 μg/kg/min, with the rate of the infusion adjusted according to the therapeutic response.

Subsequent management: Subsequent management is determined by the response to treatment, which is assessed through the continuous monitoring of the severity of asthma. Patients who respond poorly and require intensive care will be recognized and treated accordingly. As improvement is achieved the emphasis shifts to the investigation of the causes and circumstances of the severe attack, and arrangements are made for management following discharge, short- and long-term treatment, the institution of a self-management plan, and appropriate follow-up arrangements.

Further monitoring: Medical personnel should remain with the patient after initial treatment has started, or at least until clear improvement is seen. The patient should be assessed regularly, with measurement of PEFR and heart rate. The frequency of these measurements will be dictated by the response—at least every 15 minutes initially. Once improvement has occurred, a suitable regimen would include monitoring these measurements before and after bronchodilator treatment. If the patient has features of a potentially life-threatening attack, or if the patient's condition has not improved, then a repeat measurement of arterial blood-gas tension within two hours of starting treatment is also indicated.

Good response to initial treatment: If the patient's condition improves, then oxygen should be continued and nebulized β-agonists should be given every two to four hours. Oral steroids are continued throughout the admission. Because the anti-inflammatory effects of oral steroids persist for over 24 hours, once daily dosage is insufficient. In order to reduce the degree of adrenal suppression, prednisone should be given as a single dose in the morning. Treatment with inhaled anti-inflammatory treatment should be continued throughout the admission to avoid the confusion of stopping and repeatedly restarting regular treatment. If intravenous aminophylline was given initially, this may be stopped or changed to administration by the oral route, with the dose determined with the aid of measurement of plasma theophylline concentrations.

A number of treatments are contraindicated or considered to be unhelpful in the treatment of severe asthma. The prescription of sedatives has been associated with sudden death, because of their effect in reducing respiratory drive and alertness, and these are therefore contraindicated outside the intensive care unit. Antibiotics need not be given routinely, but rather prescribed where there is a specific evidence of a bacterial infection. Percussive physiotherapy is likely to distress a severely ill asthmatic patient, and is contraindicated in the initial stages, although relaxation techniques to achieve control over the rate, depth, and pattern of breathing may be helpful in the recovery phase.

Poor response to initial treatment: If repeat assessment indicates that the patient has not improved after 15 to 30 minutes, then nebulization of a β-agonist should be repeated. A regimen in which the β-agonist is administered by nebulization every 15 to 30 minutes for 60 to 90 minutes may be followed. Although the evidence is conflicting, in this situation ipratropium bromide may provide significant additional bronchodilation beyond that due to a β-agonist alone and may be added to the nebulizer solution in a dose of 0.5 mg. High-flow oxygen should be administered continuously, as severe hypoxia frequently persists even after clinical improvement. Consideration should also be given to the intravenous administration of aminophylline or a β-agonist, as outlined above.

In these patients, further investigations may be required in addition to the frequent recording of PEFR, heart rate, and repeated arterial blood-gas tensions. Urgent chest radiography should be undertaken to rule out complications such as collapse and pneumothorax. The serum potassium should be measured, particularly in patients with prior corticosteroid or diuretic treatment. Hypokalemia, due primarily to high-dose β-agonist therapy, is not uncommon in severe asthma and may require potassium supplementation. Other investigations include a full blood count and, in older patients, electrocardiography.

Indication for intensive care and assisted ventilation: Patients with features of potentially life-threatening asthma who are not responding to treatment or those with features suggesting that they are at imminent risk of death should be admitted to an intensive care unit. Not all of these patients will need ventilation; however, their transfer to the intensive care unit will ensure that each is intensively monitored and can be ventilated without delay should the need arise. The indications for ventilation include patients with drowsiness, unconsciousness, or exhaustion; those with arterial blood-gas measurements indicating persistent and worsening respiratory failure; and those with a respiratory cardiac arrest.

Because the prognosis for patients with severe asthma receiving assisted ventilation is so much better when it is instituted electively before rather than following an arrest, assisted ventilation should be undertaken electively if possible. When it is undertaken, mechanical ventilation should be used to obtain the correction of hypoxemia with hyperoxic gas mixtures without attempting to restore adequate alveolar ventilation. The respirator is adjusted to avoid high airway pressures, which appear to be more dangerous than persistent hypercapnia even with $PaCO_2$ values of up to

90 mmHg. With this regimen, the risks of barotrauma and cardio-respiratory failure, both frequent fatal complications, are significantly decreased. Correction of hypercapnia is obtained later when relief of bronchial obstruction occurs. Characteristically, a volume-cycled ventilator is used, using a low respiratory frequency (6 to 10 cycles per min) and a tidal volume of 8 to 12 mL/kg. The fractional concentration of oxygen in inspired air is adapted to obtain a PaO_2 of >70 mmHg. Ventilation is adapted in order to achieve the optimal volume per minute compatible with maximum peak inspiratory airway pressures of <50 cm H_2O.

It has been shown that the best ventilatory parameter to predict the development of complications such as hypotension and barotrauma is the end inspiratory lung volume above functional residual capacity (VEI), a measurement of dynamic hyperinflation. As a result of these findings, an alternative mechanical ventilatory regimen has been recommended in which ventilation is adapted to achieve a VEI of <1.4 L, with initial ventilation settings for a tidal volume of 8 to 10 mL/kg; inspiratory flow of 80 to 100 L/min, and rate 11 to 14 breaths per minute, to achieve an initial ventilation of <115 mL/kg/min. The VEI is then measured as soon as possible and repeated regularly with ventilator adjustments made to ensure that the VEI remains <1.4 L (or <20 mL/kg).

If ventilatory support is undertaken, patients need to be sedated and paralyzed. Pancuronium and a benzodiazepine are recommended as they both lack mast cell degranulating effects and cause minimal depression of blood pressure and cardiac output. The role of intravenous bicarbonate to prevent the adverse effects of acidosis is uncertain.

Predischarge considerations—circumstances associated with the exacerbation: The events leading up to the admission need to be reviewed in detail in an attempt to identify factors which led to the attack being of sufficient severity to warrant a hospital admission. Particular emphasis should be placed on the recognition by the patient of his or her deteriorating asthma and on whether the patient's therapeutic response was appropriate. The patient's long-term maintenance of treatment should be reviewed, and an attempt made to identify avoidable precipitating causes. In discussion of the problems associated with self-management of the attack requiring hospital admission, the opportunity exists to introduce a self-management plan along the lines outlined above.

Duration of hospital admission: The duration of the hospital admission following a severe asthmatic attack cannot be rigidly set, as it will depend on the individual patient and the available resources. Ideally, before leaving the hospital patients should be clinically stable with no nocturnal symptoms and with PEFR consistently >75% of their best levels and diurnal variability of <25%. The rationale for these criteria is based on studies that have shown that patients discharged from the hospital before they reach this level are of an increased risk of a severe attack requiring re-admission and that marked peak flow variability in the hospital is associated with sudden asthma death. Thus it is recommended that discharge be delayed until stable PEFR values are achieved. At least 24 hours prior to scheduled discharge, the patient should be changed from nebulized to his or her routine aerosol or dry-powdered metered-dose inhaler to ensure that clinical stability is maintained on this lower dose of β-agonist.

Guided self-management: The institution of an asthma self-management plan provides guidance relating to discharge medications. A patient should continue on a high dose of oral steroids until the asthma is fully stable and optional lung function is achieved before reducing the dose. This may well require the use of oral corticosteroids for a period of up to two to three weeks. Although this may lead to hypothalamic–pituitary–adrenal axis suppression, this recovers within a few days, and patients are able to mount a normal adrenal response to stress during the recovery period. Relapse requiring readmission is more likely to occur in patients who do not take steroids following discharge.

All patients should be discharged on regular inhaled anti-inflammatory treatment—for most, this will be an inhaled corticosteroid at a higher dose than that taken before admission. In fact, there is probably sufficient evidence to recommend that any patient who has experienced an episode of severe asthma requiring hospital admission should receive high-dose inhaled corticosteroids (>1000 µg/day beclomethasone dipropionate or budesonide) regularly for at least six months afterwards. Patients should also have an inhaled β-agonist for use as required to relieve episodes of symptomatic bronchoconstriction. Every patient should have a peak flow meter and a written management plan showing how to modify treatment according to changes in symptoms, peak flow rate, and response to inhaled bronchodilator drugs.

Follow-up arrangements: The follow-up after discharge is an important component of management, and an appointment with the primary-care physician within a week of discharge is recommended. By virtue of their hospital admission, these patients have identified themselves as a group at considerably increased risk of subsequent morbidity and mortality. For this reason, a case could be made for all such patients to have initial follow-up with a specialist as well as the primary-care physician, an approach that has been shown to result in a reduction in morbidity. As asthmatic patients become increasingly familiar with their own self-management, their requirement for intensive medical supervision decreases.

SELECTED REFERENCES

Corbridge TC, Hall JB. The assessment and management of adults with status asthmaticus. Am J Respir Crit Care Med 1995;151:1296–1316.

D'Souza W, Crane J, Burgess C, et al. Community-based asthma care: trail of a "credit card" asthma self-management plan. Eur Respir J 1994;7:1260–1265.

International Consensus Report on Diagnosis and Treatment of Asthma. National Heart, Lung and Blood Institute, National Institutes of Health, Bethesda, MD, 1992. Clin Exp Allergy 1992;22:Suppl 1.

Manthous CA. Management of severe exacerbations of asthma. Am J Med 1995;99:298–308.

Nocturnal Asthma

9

BACKGROUND

Worsening of symptoms or decrements in airway function frequently occur in the asthmatic population during sleep. In a survey of 7729 asthmatic patients in the United Kingdom, 94% responded that they awoke at least one night a month with symptoms of asthma. Seventy-four percent awoke at least one night a week, 64% at least three nights a week, and 39% awoke every night (Table 9-1). The occurrence of these symptoms is also reflected in mortality statistics. For all age groups, 53% of asthma mortality cases over a one-year period occurred at night. Of these, 79% had had complaints of asthma affecting their sleep, and this occurred every night in 42%. Further, 94% of dyspneic episodes in patients occurred between 10 P.M. and 7 A.M., with the peak at 4 A.M. Thus, the incidence of this potentially serious problem is higher than previously realized.

MECHANISMS OF NOCTURNAL ASTHMA

Much attention has been directed at determining the mechanism of this frequent and potentially fatal clinical problem (Figure 9-1). Sixty-eight percent of deaths attributed to asthma occur between midnight and 8 A.M. This suggests that a subgroup of asthmatic patients may have impaired arousal to important stimuli. This blunted arousal may be more important among older asthmatics as they buffer a markedly higher proportion of asthma deaths.

In another investigation, sleep following sleep deprivation produced a doubling in airway resistance before the subjects awoke complaining of chest tightness and/or wheezing, compared to the

Table 9-1. Frequency of Nocturnal Asthma

Frequency	Percent affected
Every night	39
At least 3 nights/week	64
At least 1 night/week	74

Adapted from Turner-Warwick M. Epidemiology of nocturnal asthma. Am J Med 1988;85(1B):6–8.

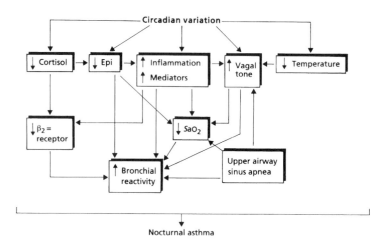

Figure 9-1. Potential Mechanisms Involved in Nocturnal Asthma. Reproduced by permission from Martin RJ. Nocturnal asthma—an overview. In: Martin RJ, ed. Nocturnal Asthma. Armonk, New York: Futura Publishing Company, 1992:101.

"normal" sleep night. Thus, arousal responses are depressed by prior sleep deprivation. In patients whose asthma is progressing over time, worsening sleep patterns probably develop that can lead to sleep deprivation and blunted arousal mechanisms.

In a survey of respiratory arrests occurring in hospitals, the crisis period was during the sleep hours between midnight and 6 A.M. A feature common to all of these patients was the presence of large circadian swings in peak expiratory flow rates (PEFR) with an early morning fall. This early morning decrease was not limited to the patient with an impending respiratory arrest; in fact, it was seen in approximately 30% of all admissions. However, PEFR swings correlated best out of all the variables analyzed with the risk of ventilatory arrest and also with sudden death.

The understanding of the pathophysiology of nocturnal asthma brings forth the important topic of chronobiology. This is the understanding of biologic processes that have time-related rhythms. These rhythms may occur yearly, monthly, or on a 24-hour cycle. For asthma, the 24-hour (circadian) cycle is extremely important.

In the normal population, the best lung-function levels occur at approximately 4 P.M. and the worst at 4 A.M. The peak-to-trough difference is approximately 8%, which is not clinically significant. For the asthmatic patient, the peak-to-trough swing can be as much as 50%. When this variation approaches 50%, it is an important indicator for potential respiratory arrest and mortality.

It has been determined that recumbency is not the factor producing the sleep-related fall in pulmonary function. Further investigations of shift workers showed that the circadian variation in peak flow is related to sleep rather than to the clock hour.

To further determine the effect of sleep on asthma, the effect of sleep interruption and sleep deprivation has been investigated. Overall, there was no significant change in early morning peak flow resulting from the interruption of sleep at 2 A.M. An important point that this aspect of the study revealed was that the fall in peak expiratory flow was often well established by 2 A.M., with progressive deterioration to 6 A.M.

Arousal does not alter the continuous drop in PEFR experienced throughout the night. The question of whether sleep itself is the causative factor in the decremental changes of expiratory flow has not been completely resolved. The relationship, at best, is complex, and it would be difficult to construct experiments that could alter the time of sleep without affecting the phase of the peak expiratory flow rhythm as well. In asthma, there is a circadian rhythm of airway resistance (increased at night) that sleep potentiates. This potentiation of resistance is related to how long one sleeps and not to sleep stages.

Bronchial hyperreactivity is a hallmark of asthma, and nocturnal worsening of lung function implies increasing reactivity during sleep. The greater the overnight fall in PEFR, the larger the circadian change in bronchial reactivity. When bronchial reactivity is tested at 4 P.M. and 4 A.M., a marked increase in reactivity occurs at 4 A.M. In addition, increased circadian variation in PEFR is related to the bronchial reactivity to histamine (tested between noon and 5 P.M.) and the response to an inhaled β_2-agonist.

The change in bronchial reactivity could affect or be affected by a variety of factors. The decrease in serum cortisol, circulating epinephrine, and cyclic AMP, as well as an increase in histamine, during the night could have a direct effect on the airways as well as an interactive effect with bronchial reactivity. Similarly, cholinergic tone, which increases at night, could affect bronchial responsivity and produce nocturnal effects. Gastroesophageal reflux and airway cooling, both of which can increase vagal tone, may induce nocturnal worsening of lung function in asthma, particularly when airway reactivity is increased. Finally, the demonstration that neutrophils and eosinophils in bronchoalveolar lavage fluid are increased at 4 A.M. in patients with nocturnal worsening of asthma, but not in those without nocturnal worsening, suggests that airway inflammation may contribute to the increase in bronchial reactivity.

Nocturnal awakenings in asthmatics occur more frequently from REM sleep, and oxygen desaturation with irregular non-apneic breathing is also worse during this stage (Table 9-2).

Mild isocapnic hypoxia (oxygen saturation about 87%) during daytime studies significantly increases bronchial responsiveness to aerosolized methacholine in mild asthmatic patients. Further investigation is needed in regard to the potential of hypoxia as a contributor to the nocturnal worsening of lung function in asthma.

Sleep apnea and nocturnal asthma

Since sleep apnea occurs in approximately 2 to 5% of the general population, one would expect to find a subset of patients that have both obstructive apnea and asthma. These patients additionally have symptoms of sleep apnea with heavy snoring during sleep. It was

---

Table 9-2. Sleep Stages and Respiratory Patterns in Nocturnal Asthma

I. Sleep stages

Increases in airway resistance during the night are related to duration of sleep and not sleep stages.

II. Respiratory patterns

A. Hypopneas and/or prolongation of expiration (reflecting increased airway resistance) are most frequent abnormalities.

B. Apneas—not frequent occurrences
  1. Central
  2. Upper airway obstruction
  3. Mixed

Adapted from Martin RJ. Cardiorespiratory disorders during sleep. Armonk, NY: Futura Publishing Company, 1984.

noted that this sonorous snoring started prior to the onset of the unstable asthma in most patients. Of great interest was the finding that nasal continuous positive airway pressure (CPAP) significantly improved both the morning and evening PEFR pre- and postinhaled bronchodilator. Additionally, although the post–nasal CPAP two-week evaluation showed a decline in PEFR, there continued to be a beneficial effect on the asthma compared to the initial baseline period.

Patients with obstructive sleep apnea and coexisting asthma can be safely treated with nasal CPAP therapy. Perhaps of greater interest and importance is that the relief of the sleep apnea in some manner not only improves the asthma during the night, but also has a carryover daytime effect. The mechanism(s) by which this occurs is (are) not known, although use of nasal CPAP may stabilize the upper airway and remove the chronic nightly irritation to the oropharyngeal area, with subsequent elimination of the reflex bronchoconstriction.

Exposure to bedding or room allergens, particularly house dust, is a simple and attractive explanation for sleep-related asthma, but does not explain the vast majority. Alternatively, exposure to certain antigens during the day can result in late-phase (delayed) bronchospasm many hours later. This may correspond to the nocturnal hours in some patients. It now appears that the time of day that the patient is exposed to the antigen is very important in determining if a late asthmatic response will occur. An evening allergen exposure can lead to the late asthmatic response in almost 100% of sensitive individuals. This then can lead to severe nocturnal bronchoconstriction.

Asthma is a disease of the airways, and this includes all airways, both intrathoracic and extrathoracic. Chronic sinusitis and/or postnasal drip are frequent problems in asthmatics. The exact reason for worsening of symptoms in asthmatics because of sinus problems or extrathoracic secretions is not known. One possibility is a nasal or laryngeal irritation reflex producing bronchoconstriction. If nasal congestion is present and the patient is mouth breathing, worsening of nocturnal symptoms may develop. A third possibility is that these secretions are aspirated, which can set off direct or reflex mechanisms worsening the asthma. Gastroesophageal reflux may be a factor in nocturnal asthma; the gastric contents irritate the esophageal mucosa and a reflex bronchoconstriction may occur via the vagal system. Several surgical reports relate that gastroesophageal reflux with possible tracheobronchial aspiration is a trigger factor in asthma. The predominant mechanism initiating the condition identified in these reported cases was an incompetent lower esophageal sphincter with or without an associated hiatal hernia. The medications with which asthmatics are treated (e.g., bronchodilators and steroids) tend to cause or potentiate the decreased tone in the gastroesophageal sphincter. The cause and effect of reflux asthma were stated to occur in several of these reports when asthmatic symptoms were abolished following the surgical restoration of effective lower esophageal sphincter function. The entire area of gastroesophageal reflux with and without aspiration needs further investigation to determine the exact relationship between reflux and asthma.

A fall in body temperature of $0.7°C$ secondary to a short-duration cold exposure produces acute asthma attacks in the majority of asthmatic patients. Since body temperature can normally decrease by approximately $1°C$ during sleep, this could be a potential mechanism of nocturnal asthma. Breathing warm, humidified air improves, but does not eliminate, the overnight decrement in lung function. Although breathing warm, humidified air may produce improvement in the overnight lung function of many asthmatic patients, caution is needed as some asthmatics may have exacerbation of symptoms by either heat or humidification.

Heightened vagal activity at night may be of importance in patients with nocturnal asthma. High-dose inhaled anticholinergic agents taken at night have been shown to reduce nocturnal asthma to varying degrees.

The effects of the vagus nerve may be enhanced during the night in asthma by upregulation of the muscarinic receptors due to inflammation and mediator release seen at night. This may also exaggerate the effects of the normal circadian variation in vagal tone.

There appears to be a temporal relationship between the nadir of circadian catecholamine and pulmonary function levels. The low point for either urinary or plasma catecholamine levels is between 3 A.M. and 4 A.M. This may be of importance, as a fall in circulating epinephrine could directly reduce the stimulation of β-adrenergic receptors in bronchial smooth muscle, inducing bronchospasm. In addition, an indirect effect of a decrease in circulating epinephrine is the release of histamine from mast cells because of diminished stimulation of β-adrenergic receptors. This is important as histamine levels in venous plasma can correlate with the degree of bronchospasm.

There is a significant increase in bronchoalveolar lavage fluid inflammatory cells in patients with asthma whose lung function is worse during sleep. Neutrophils and eosinophils increase while lymphocytes and epithelial sloughing appear to be more prominent in these subjects at 4 A.M. These changes are not related to differences in sleep pattern as much as to sleep efficiency and sleep staging. These circadian alterations in bronchoalveolar lavage fluid total cells, neutrophils, and eosinophils are not apparent in the peripheral leukocyte counts. It is possible that the inflammatory changes and epithelial damage result in increased bronchial reactivity and play an important role in the production of nocturnal asthma.

Corticosteroid levels

Multiple investigators have attempted to establish a relationship between circadian variations in airway caliber and plasma cortisol. The nadir of plasma cortisol occurs at midnight while the PEFR trough was at 4 A.M. At a physiologic dose range, hydrocortisone does not abolish airways inflammation and the development of nocturnal asthma. In pharmacologic doses, corticosteroid infusion during sleep resulted in greater than 40% improvement in the overnight decrement in FEV_1. These results emphasize the contribution of corticosteroid-sensitive factors to nocturnal worsening of asthma in a setting of clinically stable daytime symptoms and in spite of daytime therapy with corticosteroids. This observation suggests that, in addition to dose, timing of corticosteroid therapy may be important in achieving optimal effectiveness in managing nocturnal asthma.

β_2-adrenergic receptors

In general, asthmatic patients have been shown to have lower leukocyte β-adrenergic receptor density in the morning compared with daytime measurements. The reason for the altered β_2-receptor data has not been elucidated. Various physiologic conditions can regulate transmembrane signaling elements. The interaction between β-adrenergic receptor and adenylate cyclase is an example. The β-adrenergic receptor can be upregulated with glucocorticoids (or, conversely, downregulated by decreased levels) and downregulated by β-agonists through regulation of receptor mRNA.

The exact cause of nocturnal exacerbation of asthma is far from understood. More than likely, a combination of multiple

163

effects controls the airways of susceptible patients (see Figure 9-1). These processes would include the net effect of catecholamines, β-adrenergic receptor responsiveness, mucociliary clearance, reflux mechanisms, vagal tone, inflammation/mediators, corticosteroids, immunologic integrity, and arousal patterns. It appears that the circadian rhythms of all these factors are arranged to increase the potential for nocturnal bronchoconstriction, respiratory failure, and death.

THERAPY

The treatment of nocturnal asthma—and, actually, asthma in general—is based on the understanding of the circadian rhythms and the appropriate knowledge of how each medication truly works. Thus chronopharmacology is the appropriate approach—that is, directing more intense therapy to when the disease is the worse (Table 9-3).

Potentially reversible factors

One should always approach the problem of treating nocturnal asthma by attempting to rule out any reversible causative factors. Investigation into the possibility of an intrinsic causative agent, particularly in the work environment, should be considered. Even if the patient is asymptomatic during the day, nocturnal exacerbation of asthma can be seen as a delayed effect. Be certain that the patient is not sleeping with the family dog or cat, an unfortunate but common environmental "agent." Another factor is the origin of secretions, whether intra- or extrathoracic. If the asthmatic patient also has a degree of bronchitis or bronchiectasis, decreased

---

Table 9-3. Management of Nocturnal Asthma

- Allergen avoidance
- If sleep apnea present, nasal CPAP
- If sinusitis present, treat with antibiotics, possibly nasal steroids
- If gastroesophageal reflux present, H_2 blockers, proton pump inhibitors, elevate head of bed, no bedtime snacks
- Long-acting β_2-agonists
- Sustained-release theophylline, dose timed to have peak effect during sleep
- Corticosteroid; if given orally, dose at ~3 P.M.
- Consider inhaled anticholinergics

---

clearance associated with sleep can worsen the problem. Bronchial hygiene, including postural drainage and percussion during the day and before sleep, has been beneficial in occasional patients. Asthmatics commonly have sinusitis, nasal congestion, and accumulation of secretions in the posterior pharynx. This causes poor sleep and can contribute to nocturnal asthma. Correcting this with oral decongestants, nasal steroid preparations, and saline nasal washes can greatly improve the nocturnal asthma in this subset of patients. If antibiotics are needed, then three weeks of therapy is indicated due to the poor circulation in the sinus area. Rarely, a surgical procedure needs to be done to correct a particularly difficult-to-control sinus condition.

Sleep apnea: As discussed above, if the asthmatic patient also has sleep apnea, then nasal CPAP can produce beneficial bronchodilator effects for correction during both the night and day.

Reflux: Gastroesophageal reflux may or may not play an important role in nocturnal exacerbations. Aspiration should be considered and treatment based on the clinical condition. However, treatment may not improve the nocturnal asthma.

Pharmacologic interventions

The majority of patients will not benefit from the above therapeutic interventions and will need some form of bronchodilator/anti-inflammatory therapy. This may include simply maximizing a subtherapeutic program to ensure optimal bronchodilatory effects throughout the entire 24-hour day or additional maneuvers. These additional processes would be changes in the program of oral or inhaled agents. Inhaled agents are usually short-lived and do not give therapeutic effects throughout the entire night. However, an occasional patient may have difficulty only at the two to three hour mark after sleep onset. In this situation, optimal inhaled treatments at bedtime can improve the sleep period.

β_2-**Adrenergic agonists:** Salmeterol, a long-acting β-agonist, is now available in the United States. This agent has a duration of action up to 12 hours and thus is particularly useful for controlling nocturnal symptoms. Currently, only studies in patients with relatively mild decrements in lung function have been carried out using these agents. These studies have the mild overnight decrements in lung function. Studies have demonstrated that β-

adrenergic receptor function decreases at night in patients with the nocturnal worsening of their asthma, and this may indicate that higher doses of β_2-agents are needed during the night. In a group of asthmatic subjects with and without nocturnal asthma, salmeterol, in doses of $50\,\mu g$ and $100\,\mu g$ inhaled twice daily, resulted in an overall improvement in morning PEFR compared to a placebo.

Theophylline: One study has shown the superiority of a sustained-released theophylline preparation in treating asthmatics with mild to moderate nocturnal asthma compared to an intermediate inhaled β_2-agonist. In this study it is important to note that sleep quality and architecture were unchanged between the various preparations, demonstrating that the presence of theophylline did not alter sleep compared to the β_2-agonist. Additionally, not only was the FEV_1 improved in the morning, but there was less nocturnal oxygen desaturation while on theophylline.

In subjects with more significant nocturnal asthma, higher serum theophylline concentrations (STC) during the night and lower STC during the daytime, where it is easier to control the bronchoconstriction, have been demonstrated to be successful. Higher STC (about $16\,\mu g/ml$) from 3 A.M. to 5 A.M. produced a marked improvement in the overnight worsening of lung function versus lower therapeutic levels (about $11.5\,\mu g/ml$). During the daytime the STC of 9 to 14 $\mu g/ml$ produced the same bronchodilator effect on the FEV_1. Another study also showed a significant relationship between increasing STC and improvement in FEV_1 from 2 A.M. to 6 A.M., but not from 2 P.M. to 6 P.M. Also, it helps to explain why previous studies on theophylline occurring during the daytime have not shown that increasing the serum theophylline concentration above approximately $10\,\mu g/ml$ improves lung function any further. Furthermore, sleep quality and architecture are not altered between higher and lower therapeutic STC, but there is less oxygen desaturation with higher STC.

Corticosteroids: Another example of chronopharmacology would involve the use of corticosteroids. If an asthma patient needs steroids, then every effort should be made to use inhaled steroids. If oral steroids are needed for long periods of time, every other day would be preferable to every morning. However, there are many steroid-dependent asthmatics with nocturnal asthma. An important fact to consider is that increasing a steroid dose by ten-fold will increase the length of action only by two-fold. As a result, increasing the morning dose in these individuals usually leads to more steroid complications without improvement in nighttime asthma control. Consideration of the use of an afternoon dose should be undertaken. Since the nocturnal worsening of asthma is associated with an increase in inflammation and mediator release, it would be reasonable to assume that therapy directed at this aspect would be of benefit. Studies have begun to clarify the contribution of timing of corticosteroids to their ability to block the circadian recruitment of inflammatory cells into the lung. The data highlight the relevance of prednisone dose timing in attenuating the nocturnal worsening of asthmatic lung function and decrement in airways inflammation. A 3 P.M. dose produced significant improvement in overnight spirometry (placebo control, $-28\% \pm 7\%$; steroid, -10% $\pm 4\%$) as well as a sustained reduction of blood eosinophils during both the early evening and the sleep-related hours. Additionally, the 3 P.M. dose of prednisone produced a pancellular reduction in the 4 A.M. bronchoalveolar lavage cytology. These effects were not demonstrated with either an 8 A.M. or 8 P.M. dose phase. Neither alternative time produced an improvement in overnight spirometry or reduction in any bronchoalveolar lavage cellular profile. Alterations in blood eosinophil number by the 8 A.M. and 8 P.M. phases suggest that eosinophil recruitment or activation occurs prior to spirometric decline.

Overall, the results suggest that the 3 P.M. dose of prednisone interrupts the inflammatory cascade at one or more critical steps in its genesis. Thus, oral steroids, if needed, should be given at this time of day. Corticosteroids are known to influence both the function and kinetics of all the inflammatory cells represented in the bronchoalveolar lavage. It has been demonstrated that elevations in total white cell number and neutrophil, eosinophil, and lymphocyte counts in the bronchoalveolar lavage fluid of the nocturnal asthma cohort when compared to asthmatics without nocturnal worsening. These observations support a collaborative cellular mechanism of inflammation which is corticosteroid-sensitive, yet dependent on timing in addition to dosage.

The use of inhaled steroids is of interest in patients with nocturnal asthma. One would think that these agents would be ideal for this problem. However, studies have given mixed results. One study showed that in 14 asthmatic patients with nocturnal symptoms and morning decreases in PEFR, only eight patients resolved the nocturnal component using inhaled beclomethasone (or inhaled albuterol). The dose of beclomethasone was higher than standard, 400 μg four times per day. Although the other six patients improved in daytime lung function, the overnight decrements in function did not improve. The reason for this interesting finding is not immediately apparent, but certainly needs further investigation.

Anticholinergics: Vagal tone is increased at night. Unfortunately, there is no anticholinergic of long enough duration presently available if this form of therapy is selected. Ipratropium bromide, a currently available anticholinergic bronchodilator, is usually given at two puffs (40 μg) per dose. Higher bedtime dosing (80 μg) compared to the usual daytime dosing is needed to lengthen the duration of effective action of the drug. If the patient wakes during the night, then inhalation of ipratropium bromide can be of great benefit if given in sufficient doses at bedtime.

CONCLUSION

Indeed, the sleeping patient is still a patient, and it is of utmost importance that clinicians understand the circadian and sleep-related events that occur. To neglect this area of medicine hinders the care of the patient and accelerates the disease process.

SELECTED REFERENCES

Beam WR, Weiner DE, Martin RJ. Timing of prednisone and alterations of airway inflammation in nocturnal asthma. Am Rev Respir Dis 1992:1524–1530.

Jarjour NN, Busse WW, Calhoun WJ. Enchanced production of oxygen radicals in nocturnal asthma. Am Rev Respir Dis 1992;146:905–911.

Martin RJ, Cicutto LC, Smith HR, et al. Airway inflammation in nocturnal asthma. Am Rev Respir Dis 1991;143:351–377.

Oosterhoff Y, Tineus W, Postma DS. The role of airway inflammation in the pathophysiology of nocturnal asthma. Clin Exp Allergy 1995;25:915–921.

Pincus DJ, Beam WR, Martin RJ. Chronobiology and chronotherapy of asthma. Clin Chest Med 1995;16:699–713.

Aspirin-sensitive Asthma

10

INTRODUCTION

Aspirin and related compounds are categorized as nonsteroidal anti-inflammatory drugs (NSAIDs). These agents share the property of inhibiting cyclooxygenase, an important enzyme in the metabolic pathway of arachidonic acid (Figure 10-1). These medications have anti-inflammatory effects, which make them important for the treatment of rheumatological conditions, are antipyretic, and have analgesic properties. In addition, aspirin is widely used for its ability to prevent platelet aggregation. A listing of some of the available nonsteroidal anti-inflammatory drugs can be found in Table 10-1.

ADVERSE REACTIONS

Adverse reactions to aspirin and other NSAIDs are not uncommon. Gastrointestinal upset and peptic ulceration are well-known complications. These medications have been known to decrease renal function, which may in turn lead to edema and weight gain. Intoxication due to an overdose of aspirin can result in headache, dizziness, tinnitus, hearing impairment, central nervous system disturbances, and metabolic acidosis.

Idiosyncratic reactions may occur in certain patients. Patients with systemic lupus erythematosus or mixed connective-tissue disease may develop a hypersensitivity reaction consisting of fever, abdominal pain, nausea, vomiting, and abnormalities of liver function, associated with fatty changes on liver biopsy.

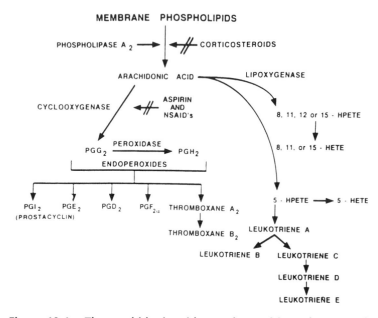

Figure 10-1. The arachidonic acid cascade. Aspirin and nonsteroidal anti-inflammatory drugs inhibit the enzyme cyclooxygenase. Corticosteroids inhibit the action of phospholipase A_2. Reprinted from Busse WW, Holgate ST. Asthma and Rhinitis. Boston: Blackwell Science, 1995.

Occasionally patients may experience adverse reactions to aspirin and NSAIDs that mimic allergic reactions. Some people may experience urticarial reactions or angioedema on exposure to aspirin. Others may develop life-threatening anaphylactoid reactions. These patients are otherwise normal. To date no evidence for an IgE-mediated reaction has been recognized.

A subgroup of patients with chronic urticaria may also note exacerbations of their hives and angioedema with ingestion of aspirin or NSAIDs. These patients typically tolerate aspirin and NSAIDs before the development of their chronic urticaria. The pathogenesis of this condition is not known but obviously represents an acquired situation.

In addition to the cutaneous and systemic reactions to aspirin and nonsteroidal NSAIDs, respiratory reactions may also occur. These may affect both the upper and lower respiratory passages. Since the 1920s, aspirin and NSAIDs have become well recognized as a cause of acute bronchoconstriction and potentially fatal asthma. Finally, an association of aspirin sensitivity, asthma, and nasal polyps has long been recognized.

Table 10-1. Nonsteroidal Anti-inflammatory Drugs

Acidic	Enolic acids	Nonacidic
Carboxylic acids	Oxicams	Naphthylakanoes
Fernamic acids e.g.,	e.g., piroxicam,	e.g.,
meclofenamate sodium,	sudoxicam,	nulaumetone,
flufenamic acid, mefenamic	tenoxicam,	proquazone,
acid, niflumic acid	isoxicam	bufexamac
Acetic acids	Pyrazolones	
e.g., sulindac, indomethacin,	e.g.,	
tolmetin, diclofenac	phenylbutazone,	
Pyranocarboxylic acids e.g.,	oxyphenbutazone	
etodolac, ketorolac		
Propionic acids		
e.g., naproxen sodium,		
flurbiprofen, ibuprofen,		
ketoprofen, fenoprofen,		
pirprofen, indoprofen,		
tiaprofenic, oxaprozin,		
fenbuten, carprofen, suprofen		
Salicylic acids		
Acetylated e.g., aspirin		
Non-acetylated e.g., salsalate,		
diflunisal, choline salicylate,		
salicylate, salicylamicly		
sodium salicylate		

A classification of respiratory responses to aspirin and NSAIDs based on provocative challenges has been devised. These patterns of adverse reactions can be categorized as follows:

1. A positive asthmatic response. These individuals experience a decline in FEV_1 values of ≥25% below the baseline.
2. A partial asthmatic response. These individuals experience a decline in FEV_1 of ≥15%, but ≤25% from the baseline value.
3. Naso–ocular response. These patients experience a profound reaction, limited to the nasal and ocular system, consisting of nasal congestion, rhinorrhea, and/or ocular injection with chemosis and lacrimation.
4. The classic response. These individuals experience the simultaneous occurrence of both a positive asthmatic response and naso–ocular symptoms.

5. Nonresponders. These patients have an absence of upper or lower respiratory tract symptoms and a ≤15% decline in FEV$_1$ from baseline value after ingestion of 650 mg of aspirin.

POPULATIONS AT RISK FOR ASPIRIN SENSITIVITY

No predisposing factor has been identified for the development of urticaria, angioedema, or anaphylactoid reactions. These patients are essentially normal, although some may have familial histories of reactions of this type. These patients may at times demonstrate immediate positive skin-test reactions to common aeroallergens. Peripheral blood eosinophilia has been demonstrated in some. Patients who experience worsening of their chronic urticaria during aspirin ingestion cannot be distinguished from those who do not respond.

Patients at greatest risk for aspirin sensitivity appear to be those who have underlying asthma and chronic rhinosinusitis. These are the patients with the so-called "aspirin triad." This condition typically affects women more than men, by a ratio of 3:2. The onset of rhinitis symptoms usually begins at age 20 to 40 or greater. Patients complain of a chronic rhinitis with intermittent profuse, watery rhinorrhea, and anosmia may frequently occur along with severe nasal congestion. Physical examination may demonstrate the presence of nasal polyps with a pale, congested nasal mucosa. Nasal smear will often demonstrate eosinophilia. Sinusitis occurs in over 90% of cases. Peripheral blood eosinophilia is common. Only about one-third of affected individuals appear to have IgE-mediated sensitivity to inhalant allergens as demonstrated by skin testing or by radioallergosorbent test (RAST). Bronchial asthma may subsequently follow and often becomes chronic and severe. The asthma may eventually become resistant to the usual therapeutic modalities and require corticosteroid therapy to control symptoms. At some point during this progressive illness, a patient may develop a reaction to aspirin, principally affecting the respiratory system. Urticarial reactions in these patients are decidedly uncommon. In some instances a familial clustering of cases has been observed.

Aspirin sensitivity in children is similar to that of adult patients in that there is a slight preponderance of girls who are affected compared to boys. Sinusitis is also more frequent in aspirin-sensitive asthmatic children, compared to asthmatic children who tolerate aspirin. These children also may be slightly more prone to develop steroid dependency than aspirin–tolerant asthmatics. On occasion these children may also exhibit nasal polyposis.

PREVALENCE OF ASPIRIN SENSITIVITY

The prevalence of aspirin sensitivity among various groups of patients is dependent on the method used to diagnose the condition. Provocative challenge testing conducted in patients with a history of aspirin sensitivity demonstrates a lack of response in 15 to 20%.

Nonasthmatics may occasionally develop urticaria, angioedema, or anaphylactoid reactions to aspirin, although these are rare. The estimated frequency of aspirin intolerance or sensitivity in the general population is approximately 0.3%.

For the patient with chronic urticaria whose lesions are exacerbated by aspirin and nonsteroidal anti-inflammatory drugs, the occurrence is not uncommon. Twenty to thirty percent of these individuals are aspirin intolerant.

Various estimates of the frequency of aspirin sensitivity in asthmatic patients have been reported, usually ranging between 5 and 20% of adult asthmatics. In asthmatic children less than 10 years of age, aspirin sensitivity appears to be fairly rare. In older children and young adults, age 10 to 20 years, the prevalence is estimated to be approximately 10%. In adults who only have asthma, the prevalence estimate is 10 to 20%. However, a high-risk population appears to be those with asthma, nasal polyposis, and chronic rhinosinusitis. Some 30 to 40% of these patients have demonstrable aspirin sensitivity. In patients who have asthma, chronic rhinosinusitis, and a history of an adverse reaction to aspirin, 60 to 85% respond positively on an aspirin challenge. The frequency of aspirin sensitivity in adults with only rhinosinusitis is not known, but may approach 15%. In a study of hospitalized asthmatics, 19% were found to have positive aspirin challenge.

Because of the severity of the respiratory responses that can be provoked by aspirin, physicians need to be aware of the prevalence of this condition among their asthma patients. Because of the high degree of risk for certain patient populations, instructions for the avoidance of aspirin or NSAIDs may be particularly important.

MECHANISMS OF ASPIRIN SENSITIVITY

The mechanism of aspirin sensitivity is currently unknown. A number of hypotheses have been proposed, although no single unifying concept has been established. The majority of patients with aspirin sensitivity are nonatopic but do demonstrate nasal and peripheral blood eosinophilia. To date no convincing evidence for an IgE-mediated reaction has been forthcoming.

One group of investigators has associated aspirin-sensitive asthma with the presence of the genetic phenotype HLA-DQw2. While this finding has not been confirmed by other investigators, it suggests there may be a genetic factor responsible for the development of aspirin sensitivity.

The release of the chemical mediators of anaphylaxis from mast cells and other cells through nonimmunologic mechanisms has also been hypothesized as a potential mechanism for aspirin-induced asthma. Direct evidence for a role of the mast cell and its mediators in the pathogenesis of aspirin-induced reactions was demonstrated by the development of elevated plasma histamine levels and the appearance of mast-cell tryptase in the serum of aspirin-sensitive patients undergoing aspirin challenge. These patients experienced moderate to severe respiratory reactions and had cutaneous and/or gastrointestinal involvement as well. In contrast, 14 other patients who experienced only respiratory reactions without extrapulmonary symptoms had no change in plasma tryptase or histamine levels. This suggests a potential role for the mast cell and its mediators in certain aspirin-sensitive asthmatics, but not all.

Currently the most plausible explanation for aspirin sensitivity is a biochemical defect brought about by the inhibition of cyclooxygenase. Evidence to support this hypothesis includes the fact that analgesics that inhibit cyclooxygenase precipitate bronchoconstriction in aspirin-sensitive patients while analgesics that do not affect cyclooxygenase do not produce these effects. There is a positive correlation between the potency of these drugs to inhibit cyclooxygenase in vitro and their potency to induce asthma attacks in sensitive patients. At one time it was considered that the inhibition of the cyclooxygenase pathway with the loss of prostaglandin E_2 (PGE$_2$), which has bronchodilating properties, would explain the situation. Alternatively the shift in arachidonic acid metabolism through the lipoxygenase pathway, with resultant increase in leukotriene production, could account for increased bronchoconstriction. Neither of these simple explanations has been found to be true since the loss of PGE$_2$, which acts as a bronchodilator, or the enhancement of leukotrienes, which are bronchoconstrictatory, would be expected to cause similar reactions in all asthmatic patients, not just a subpopulation.

In addition to the cyclooxygenase pathway of alterations in the lipoxygenase pathway, metabolites of arachidonic acid are of importance in aspirin sensitivity. In a group of aspirin-sensitive patients an administration of aspirin resulted in increased levels of leukotriene C_4 and histamine in the nasal secretions of patients who experience both a naso-ocular and bronchospastic reaction to aspirin. In contrast, in patients who experience only a bronchospastic reaction, no increase in LTC_4 or histamine release was detected.

The result of introducing aspirin into the nasal passages of aspirin-sensitive subjects was compared to the responses of healthy people and aspirin-insensitive asthmatics. Inhibition of PGE_2 and $PGF_{2\alpha}$ release was detected in all three groups in the nasal secretion after aspirin installation. In contrast, the patients who were aspirin sensitive had an increase in the production of sulfidopeptide leukotrienes. The results suggest that abnormal release of leukotrienes in aspirin-sensitive asthmatic patients contributes to the nasal and bronchial reaction.

Systemic generation of leukotrienes has also been studied. Urinary leukotriene E_4 levels were studied in a group of asthmatics tolerant to aspirin and asthmatics sensitive to aspirin. At baseline, the urinary leukotriene levels in the aspirin-sensitive subjects were approximately six-fold greater than those of the non-aspirin-sensitive asthmatics. Following aspirin challenge in the aspirin-sensitive patients, there was evidence of bronchoconstriction followed by four-fold increase in urinary leukotriene E_4 levels three to six hours after aspirin but not placebo challenge.

Further evidence for a role of leukotrienes in the generation of aspirin sensitivity includes the fact that aspirin-sensitive asthmatics show approximately a ten-fold increase in airway responsiveness to inhaled leukotriene E_4 compared to non-aspirin-sensitive asthmatics. Lastly, the administration of leukotriene receptor antagonists and 5-lipoxygenase inhibitors can partially inhibit the bronchoconstrictatory effect of aspirin in aspirin-sensitive patients.

The basic intercellular biochemical defect responsible for aspirin sensitivity is unknown, although certain differences in platelet and basophil function have been observed. For example, investigations into the arachidonic acid metabolism in vitro by basophils stimulated with anti-IgE showed that the incubation of basophils from aspirin-sensitive patients with aspirin resulted in a greater ratio of suppression of generation of PGE_2 compared to LTD_4 for aspirin-sensitive patients than for aspirin-tolerant patients with asthma and for normal subjects. This suggests an intrinsic defect in the metabolic pathway of the arachidonic acid cascade of these individuals. However, the mechanism of aspirin sensitivity remains to be determined.

DIAGNOSIS OF ASPIRIN SENSITIVITY

The diagnosis of aspirin sensitivity is strongly suggested by the history of an adverse response. Confirmation of the diagnosis, however, is generally based on an objective challenge test. Because no IgE-mediated mechanism has been identified, skin testing or in vitro testing for specific IgE antibodies, such as the RAST, is not applicable.

Confirmation of the diagnosis may be required in patients who are candidates for aspirin or NSAID therapy. In most instances alternative analgesics and antipruritics are available that could easily be substituted. There are some patients for whom aspirin or NSAIDs are necessary.

Before considering a diagnostic challenge with aspirin, availability of staff equipment and adjacent facilities for the potential hospitalization of patients is necessary. For patients who have had anaphylactoid reactions to aspirin, the use of a diagnostic challenge is seldom indicated. However, in patients with urticaria where the risk for a severe reaction is less, diagnostic challenges may be indicated. For these patients, antihistamine should generally be continued during the challenge procedure in order to avoid false positive reactions due to discontinuation of treatment. If patients are in remission, antihistamines are not necessary and can be withheld during the challenge procedure. The criteria for a positive test is simply the appearance of an urticarial lesion or angioedema within 24 hours after the challenge ingestion. Quantitative methods for scoring urticaria have been devised. These are based on the system for assessing thermal burns to the skin. The body surface is divided into 11 areas, each of which make up approximately 9% of the cutaneous surface. Using a scoring system of 0 to 4 in which no hives is 0 and 4 indicates that more than 50% of the area is covered with hives, an objective quantitation of urticaria in each of these areas can be assessed.

Initial challenges can usually be conducted in a single-blind fashion, in which increasing doses of aspirin are given at 8 A.M. and 10 A.M. Initial doses are 100 mg followed by 325 mg. If no response is observed in the two-hour interval after the challenge, a second day of testing is usually scheduled, in which 650 and 975 mg of aspirin are administered at the time intervals given above. Confirmatory, double-blind challenges may be conducted in which a third testing day is added, during which placebos are administered in random order along with the active aspirin challenge. Because of the evanescent nature of chronic urticaria, placebo-controlled trials are especially important to confirm a positive aspirin challenge.

For patients with asthma who require aspirin therapy and give a history of aspirin sensitivity, a diagnostic challenge may be warranted. Before embarking on this procedure, all precautions should be observed, including making sure of the availability of staff and personnel to conduct intubation of the airway and mechanical ventilation. Patients can be screened by sinus x-ray films since the vast majority of aspirin-sensitive asthmatics have evidence of chronic sinusitis. It has been estimated that the chance of a positive aspirin challenge with a normal sinus x-ray film is approximately 4%.

Because of the inherent risk of a severe asthma attack with oral challenge testing, some patients may not be appropriate for testing. These include patients with fixed airway disease and an FEV_1 of less than 1.5 liters; patients with unstable asthma, as demonstrated by an improvement in FEV_1 of greater than 20% after bronchodilator therapy; those with active asthma that are nonresponsive to corticosteroids; patients receiving β-blocker therapy; patients who have psychological or compliance problems that would preclude their ability to adhere to all aspects of the testing procedure. For patients who have unstable disease, it is important to establish control of the asthma by the prior administration of oral corticosteroids for three to ten days before the procedure. Withdrawal of certain medications could result in unstable asthma, which would lead to false positive tests. Antihistamines, cromolyn, and inhaled β-agonists are usually withheld for varying periods of time before the procedure. Theophylline and corticosteroids are usually administered the day of the procedure since these do not interfere with the testing.

A uniformly accepted protocol for aspirin challenge has not been devised. For patients who have a low degree of risk of aspirin sensitivity, a one-day challenge can be conducted (Table 10-2). For patients who have a history of more severe reactions, the testing can be conducted over a three-day period (Table 10-3). Patients should be carefully observed, and pulmonary function tests which measure the FEV_1 should be given or specific airway conductance

Table 10-2. One-Day Aspirin Challenge Protocol (Low-Risk Procedure)

1. Asthma must be in remission.
2. Patient may continue theophylline and corticosteroids.
3. Discontinue antihistamines, inhaled β-adrenergic agents, and cromolyn sodium prior to challenge.
4. Administer ASA as follows:

One-Day Aspirin Challenge

Time	Aspirin dosage (mg)	Cumulative dosage (mg)
8 A.M.	30	30
10 A.M.	60	90
12 A.M.	100	190
2 P.M.	325	515
4 P.M.	650	1165
6 P.M.	End	—

5. Monitor FEV_1 and symptoms each hour.
6. Positive responses include:
   - Partial asthmatic response: decline in FEV_1 $\geq$15%, $\leq$25%.
   - Asthmatic: decline in FEV_1 $\geq$25% from baseline.
   - Naso-ocular: profound nasal and ocular congestion, rhinorrhea.
   - "Classic": continued asthmatic and naso-ocular response.
7. If a reaction does not occur, patient is not aspirin sensitive.
8. If a positive response occurs, a placebo challenge should be done $\geq$ seven days later to confirm specificity of the response.

Modified from Lumry WR, Curd JG, Stevenson DD. Aspirin-sensitive asthma and rhinosinusitis: current concepts and recent advances. Ear Nose Throat J 1984;63:66–77.

should be determined. A positive response is a $\geq$15% decline in FEV_1 after aspirin administration.

The use of inhaled lysine-aspirin solution as a bronchoprovocation in aspirin-sensitive asthma has been described. This procedure appears to be safer than oral challenge with aspirin for the diagnosis of aspirin-sensitive asthma. Inhalation of serially doubling incremental concentrations of lysine-aspirin solution allows the construction of a dose–response curve. This procedure appears to be reproducible. The bronchoconstriction is more rapid (20 to 45 minutes) than that which occurs for oral aspirin ingestion (up to 60 minutes). This procedure may eventually provide an alternative to oral aspirin challenge.

Table 10-3. Three-Day Aspirin Challenge Protocol (High-Risk Procedure)

1. Follow same precautions and recommendations as for one-day challenge (Table 10-2).
2. Administer aspirin or placebo as follows:

Three-Day Aspirin Challenge

	Day		
Time	1	2	3
8 A.M.	Placebo	30 mg	150 mg
11 A.M.	Placebo[a]	60 mg	325 mg
2 P.M.	Placebo[b]	100 mg	650 mg

[a] May substitute tartrazine 25 mg.
[b] May substitute tartrazine 50 mg.

3. Monitor FEV_1 and symptoms each hour.
4. Positive responses include partial asthmatic, asthmatic, naso–ocular, or classic (see Table 10-2).
5. Confirmatory placebo challenge should be conducted if positive response occurs.

Modified from Lumry WR, Curd JG, Stevenson DD. Aspirin-sensitive asthma and rhinosinusitis: current concepts and recent advances. Ear Nose Throat J 1984;63:66–77.

Rechallenge variability

Aspirin sensitivity appears to be an acquired situation with variation in response to aspirin exposure over time. In a study of repeated aspirin challenges at time intervals varying from four months to six years apart, 61% of patients had no variation in the response to aspirin challenge from the initial challenge. However, 39% demonstrated variability in their response to aspirin challenge. Some patients at one point lost aspirin sensitivity, but others subsequently regained sensitivity to aspirin, returning either to nasal symptoms or to a combination of nasal and asthmatic responses. Among individuals with the classical nasal and asthmatic response, some had an improvement in their response on subsequent challenge with either isolated nasal responses or less than a 20% decline in pulmonary function after aspirin challenge. A single individual lost the asthmatic response but retained nasal response to aspirin. In a few patients there was a worsening of symptoms with increased asthma after aspirin challenge.

Refractory period

In the course of aspirin challenges an interesting phenomenon has been observed, the so-called "refractory period." The refractory period occurs for a variable length of time, during which no observable reaction to aspirin occurs following the initial response.

The refractory period lasts between two and five days, and in some patients a gradual return to sensitivity occurs in two to four days. Thus, a state of tolerance to aspirin can be induced by incremental doses of aspirin over a period of one to five days. Subsequently, as long as the patient remains on aspirin therapy, the likelihood of his or her responding to aspirin remains relatively low. Upon discontinuation of the aspirin therapy for two to seven days, the aspirin sensitivity returns.

These studies have proven very useful in establishing a method by which patients with aspirin sensitivity who need aspirin or NSAID therapy can be effectively treated.

Therapy of aspirin sensitivity

Treatment of the underlying rhinosinusitis, nasal polyps, and asthma in patients with aspirin sensitivity is no different than for any other patient. The use of antihistamines, decongestants, topical nasal steroids, antibiotics, surgical procedures, bronchodilators, and anti-inflammatory antiasthmatic medications including corticosteroids and sodium cromolyn is appropriate. In patients with a high risk for aspirin sensitivity, namely those with nasal polyposis and chronic rhinosinusitis, the most pragmatic approach is avoidance of aspirin and NSAIDs. This course would obviate severe adverse reactions in this patient population.

Certain patients may need this type of therapy (e.g., for rheumatologic or cardiovascular disease). Such patients may be candidates for diagnostic challenges and be considered for desensitization protocols. Patients who have safely ingested aspirin or NSAIDs in the previous two months are unlikely to react adversely and may be started on therapy without undergoing diagnostic challenge. On the other hand, if patients have not ingested these products within the past two months or by history have demonstrated an adverse response, diagnostic challenge with consideration for desensitization would be appropriate. If a diagnostic challenge is negative, treatment can be initiated directly. However, if a previous challenge has demonstrated a positive response, the patient should then be considered for the desensitization protocol. Because of the refractory period, patients can be slowly titrated in the dose of the aspirin or NSAID to therapeutic range and then continue on this as maintenance therapy.

Long-term aspirin administration has been evaluated in terms of its effect on asthma and chronic rhinosinusitis in aspirin-sensitive patients who have undergone aspirin desensitization. In approximately half of the patients studied in these various tests, there was some improvement in asthma as identified by reduction in antiasthma medications including daily systemic corticosteroids, bursts of corticosteroids, and inhaled corticosteroids. Other studies have failed to confirm these observations.

More dramatic effects appear to have occurred in the rhinosinusitis symptoms of these patients. Improvement in nasal symptoms and reduction in the use of topical nasal steroids took place over the period the patients received aspirin therapy. In a study of patients receiving aspirin for two to eight years, a reduction in the number of hospitalizations per year, emergency room visits, outpatient visits, number of respiratory infections requiring antibiotic therapy, need for nasal polypectomies, additional sinus procedures, and improvement in the sense of smell were compared to those for patients not taking aspirin. These studies demonstrate that aspirin therapy may be useful as an adjunctive measure to improve the rhinosinusitis of patients with known aspirin sensitivity.

Some investigators have reported that the adverse effect of aspirin on asthma can be prevented by the use of antiasthmatic medications such as sodium cromolyn, antihistamines such as clemastine, or the oral antiasthmatic compound ketotifen. However, not all patients have been completely protected, and the use of these medications for this purpose is not recommended. The recent addition of leukotriene receptor antagonists, which can inhibit the pulmonary reaction to aspirin, into clinical practice may solve the problem of aspirin-sensitive asthma.

In the case of urticaria and angioedema, aspirin desensitization has not been successful. While a transient refractory period can be demonstrated, which may last up to 36 hours, the benefit cannot in most instances be sustained.

Cross-reactivity between aspirin and other NSAIDS

Essentially, all NSAIDs are capable of evoking adverse reactions in susceptible patients. The more potent the drug is in inhibiting the cyclooxygenase pathway, the more likely an adverse response is to occur.

Of note is the fact that ophthalmic preparations containing NSAIDs may be responsible for inducing asthma attacks in sensitive patients.

Many patients with aspirin sensitivity may tolerate without difficulty very weak inhibitors of the cyclooxygenase pathway, which include acetaminophen (paracetamol), salsalate, choline magnesium trisalicylate, sodium salicylate, and methylsalicylate. However, if high doses are given ($>2\,g/day$), there may be adverse responses in some patients.

Although controversial, the yellow food dye tartrazine has been implicated as a potential cause of adverse reactions in aspirin-sensitive patients. In a report of 114 aspirin-sensitive patients challenged with tartrazine, none had an adverse reaction. The presence of aspirin sensitivity does not appear to predispose patients to sensitivity to other food dyes nor to sulfiting agents.

Finally, hydrocortisone sodium succinate and hemisuccinate have been reported to cause adverse reactions when given intravenously to aspirin-sensitive patients. These patients tolerated other corticosteroid intravenous preparations such as methylprednisolone, dexamethasone, and betamethasone without difficulty. The mechanism of this effect is not known but it has been suggested that hydrocortisone should be avoided or used with caution by patients with aspirin sensitivity.

SUMMARY

Aspirin sensitivity may affect a significant number of asthma patients. At highest risk are individuals with nasal polyps and chronic rhinosinusitis. With the increasing use of NSAIDs, such patients potentially can be exposed to medications that can cause profound adverse respiratory reactions. Strategies for these patients include avoidance of these compounds as much as possible. Where such therapy is indicated in patients who have been identified by diagnostic challenges, such patients may be candidates for desensitization protocols.

Aspirin therapy has been attempted in some of these patients and has demonstrated some improvement in the rhinosinusitis symptoms and perhaps a slight, if any, benefit in asthma.

Patients should be advised of the potential risk of NSAID therapy and instructed to avoid these compounds where possible.

Hidden sources include ophthalmic preparations and numerous over-the-counter cough and cold medications.

SELECTED REFERENCES

Christie PE, Smith C, Arm JP, Lee TH. Aspirin sensitive asthma. Clin Exp Allergy 1992;22:171–179.

Lee TH. Mechanism of aspirin sensitivity. Am Rev Respir Dis 1992;145:S34–S36.

Nasser SM, Lee TH. Aspirin-induced early and late asthmatic responses. Clin Exp Allergy 1995;25:1–3.

Pleskow WW, Stevenson DD, Mathison DA, et al. Aspirin-sensitive rhinosinusitis/asthma: spectrum of adverse reactions to aspirin. J Allergy Clin Immunol 1983;71:574–579.

Stevenson DD, Simon RA. Aspirin sensitivity: respiratory and cutaneous manifestations. In: Middleton E Jr, Reed CE, Ellis EF, et al (eds). Allergy: principles and practice. St. Louis: CV Mosby, 1988:1537–1554.

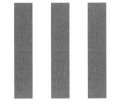

Rhinitis

Rhinitis: The Spectrum of the Disease

11

INTRODUCTION

The classification of rhinitis is troublesome for both scientist and clinician since symptoms of nasal obstruction and rhinorrhea, in combination with sneezing and an itchy feeling, are suggestive of a diagnosis of "rhinitis." Yet a whole series of mucosal afflictions can cause these symptoms. Theoretically, *rhinitis* means an inflammation of the nasal mucosa. Various classifications have been used but are often confusing because of overlapping symptoms and findings.

One may divide rhinitis into infectious, allergic, and vasomotor rhinitis. Synonyms for vasomotor rhinitis include noninfectious nonallergic rhinitis, perennial nonallergic rhinitis, and nonallergic nasal hyperreactivity with two subgroups: the eosinophilic and noneosinophilic.

More simply yet appropriately, rhinitis is either allergic or nonallergic. The allergic type can be seasonal or perennial, the nonallergic type being either infective or noninfective. Infective rhinitis may be acute or chronic, and the chronic form is either specific or nonspecific. Nonallergic noninfective rhinitis is difficult to classify and comprises vasomotor rhinitis—which is also called hyperreactive rhinitis—and conditions such as anatomical obstruction, tumors, and granulomatous disease.

The differential diagnosis of a running, stuffy, sometimes itchy nose consists of infectious, allergic, vasomotor, irritant contact, eosinophilic nonallergic, drug-induced, and hormonally induced rhinitis.

In 1978, the term *rhinopathy* was introduced to distinguish an inflammatory process (e.g., in some cases of vasomotor rhinitis).

The term rhinopathy includes six categories: atopic rhinopathy, nonatopic rhinopathy, rhinopathia vasomotoria, infectious rhinitis, polyposis nasi, and rhinitis medicamentosa.

There does not exist a uniformly accepted classification system; this is probably caused partly by overlaps among the various types of rhinitis, and partly by our lack of knowledge of the different pathophysiological phenomena.

INFECTIOUS RHINITIS
Viral causes

Rhinitis is often predominant during an upper-respiratory-tract infection. Pharyngitis, laryngitis, tracheitis, bronchitis, and conjunctivitis may accompany this rhinitis. Viral rhinitis is also called the "common cold," has an incubation period of one to four days, and usually lasts five to seven days. It can be caused by any type of virus, but rhinoviruses are the most common in adults and are considered to be the etiological organism in ±50%. Occasionally other organisms such as *Mycoplasma pneumoniae* are responsible. Thirty percent of the time no virus or other microorganism can be identified as a cause of the rhinitis. In children, rhinitis may be due to respiratory syncytial virus (RSV), additional parainfluenza viruses, or adenoviruses. The clinical picture is very common: nasal stuffiness, watery or mucoid rhinorrhea, sneezing, pain in the throat, and headache. Fever and chills are rare in adults, but more common in children. After a few days, the nasal secretions may become purulent, and cough becomes a more prominent symptom. Rhinoscopy reveals a swollen and often pale mucosa, usually with abundant secretions.

People living in crowded places or debilitated persons are more prone to viral infections. Especially for rhinoviruses, there is evidence for spreading of the disease by direct contact and not by air.

Complications are usually seen in children. Acute otitis media is the most common complication in children younger than three: 90% of the acute otitis media cases in this age group are preceded or accompanied by a viral rhinitis. In adults, acute sinusitis is usually preceded by a common cold; acute otitis media is rarer here.

To make the diagnosis of viral rhinitis, nasal secretions or a nasal washing may be collected for viral culture, but these cultures are expensive and the results are available only long after the patient has recovered. Antibody titers can be determined by the neutralization test, but need two samples: one before or at the very beginning of the infection and one three weeks after the onset of the infection. A four-fold rise in titer is suggestive for a viral infection, but here also there is too much of a time delay. An additional argument for not using antibody titers in clinical practice is the multitude of viral species.

Viruses are more effective in invading mucosa than bacteria because of their greater solubility in the mucous blanket. They bring about an exfoliation of the mucosa, which can last for weeks. Epithelial necrosis is typical with influenzal rhinitis.

Bacterial rhinitis

The normal bacterial flora of the nose includes species of corynebacteria, staphylococci, and α-hemolytic streptococci. This normal flora is an important part of the defense mechanisms of the nasal mucosa against pathogenic microorganisms.

Acute bacterial rhinitis is nearly always caused by aerobic mechanisms such as pneumococci, *Staphylococcus aureus* or *Hemophilus influenzae*. The aspect of the mucosa is smooth, red, swollen, and tender, coated with purulent secretions or, more rarely, a gray membrane of fibrin.

Bacterial rhinitis can coexist with chronic sinusitis in children and adults and with chronic adenoiditis in children. In cases of congenital unilateral choanal atresia or foreign-body rhinitis, the rhinorrhea and bacterial rhinitis are unilateral.

Bacterial superinfection is often the consequence of a common cold since the mucociliary transport mechanism is damaged. Other factors interfering with mucociliary function are cigarette smoking, cold, dryness, and some drugs.

Atrophic rhinitis

Atrophic rhinitis is characterized by a dry and crusty nasal mucosa. Ozena, in which foul-smelling crusts and secretions are present in a broadly patent nasal cavity, is the most severe degree of atrophic rhinitis. The etiology of this disease is still unknown. *Klebsiella ozaenae* has been isolated quite frequently from patients with atrophic rhinitis but is also present in other cases of purulent rhinitis. It is not understood whether this bacterium is simply an opportunistic colonizer of the injured nose or the etiologic agent of the disease. *K. ozaenae* has an inhibitory effect on cilia, which may play a potential role in pathogenesis of chronic rhinitis.

Specific infectious rhinopathies

Rhinoscleroma is an endemic disease characterized by a foul-smelling purulent rhinorrhea. Granulomatous nodules progressively grow and may result in prominence of the nostrils and upper lip. The causal organism is the gram-negative *Klebsiella rhinoscleromatis*.

In tuberculosis of the nose the causal organism is the acid-fast *Mycobacterium tuberculosis*. These patients have pain, nasal obstruction, and a bloody nasal discharge due to an isolated, ulcerated nodule on the nasal septum or inferior turbinate. Typical histological examination reveals tubercles with central necrosis.

Leprosy is an endemic disease in which the nose can become involved as part of a systemic involvement. The nasal discharge of the swollen hypersecreting mucosa is laden with *Mycobacterium leprae*. In a later state it results in crusting, bleeding, and severe obstruction.

Congenital syphilis shows purulent rhinorrhea and fissures around the anterior nares. Granulomatous destructive lesions appear in young adulthood and result in cosmetic deformity such as dorsal saddling. Acquired syphilis usually affects the nose after primary infection at other sites. According to the stage, destruction from gumma (nodular swelling on mucosa) most commonly involves the vomer and ethmoid bones. This results in progressive destruction of the nasal skeleton, with saddle deformity of the nasal dorsum and septal perforation. The causal organism is *Treponema pallidum*, which can be demonstrated by serological tests or by the presence of spirochetes in histological material from the lesions.

Fungal infection of the nose usually involves the sinuses and occurs mostly endemically (aspergillosis, rhinosporidiasis) in debilitated patients (e.g., diabetics) or patients taking immunosuppressive medication. These fungi can be cultured or demonstrated histologically. Nasal obstruction and discharge may occur but are nonspecific. In the case of mucormycosis, the organism invades along vascular channels. Arterial occlusion may result in ischemic infarction including the entire midface. In that case the prognosis is poor because of invasion of the cranium.

NONINFECTIOUS RHINITIS

Allergic rhinitis

Allergic rhinitis is a kind of inflammation of the nasal mucosa on an allergic basis. It represents a pathological state of the immune system characterized by an exaggeration of its reaction against some nonself macromolecules called allergens. "Atopic" rhinitis is a full synonym of allergic rhinitis. Following the classification of Gell and Coombs, this is a type I immediate allergic reaction that is IgE mediated.

The symptoms are sneezing, watery nasal discharge, itching, obstructed nose and sometimes eye symptoms. The aspect of the mucosa of the inferior turbinate is pale bluish. The patient can complain seasonally or perennially, although patients with the latter can show seasonal exacerbations as well. It is interesting to note that the same quantity of pollen at the end of the allergic season will aggravate the complaints (Figure 11-1).

Allergic rhinitis has a high incidence in modern populations. In the Danish population a cumulative prevalence rate of 9% was found, comparable with 10% in Michigan. Among the most common allergens we find spores (grass, trees, weeds), house dust mites, molds, and animal dander. Children of atopic parents are hereditarily predisposed to suffer an atopic disease. Children with atopic eczema or asthma have a higher chance of having allergic rhinitis. Among allergic rhinitis patients, birth in March and April was significantly overrepresented and in July underrepresented. The complaints have an early onset in life (one to twenty years) and disappear progressively during adulthood.

Mostly, the diagnosis is made by the patient's history and skin tests. Specific IgE by radioallergosorbent test (RAST) may be used as an alternative to skin tests. Total serum IgE level by RIA is not as sensitive or as specific as skin tests for diagnosis of allergic rhinitis. Counting eosinophils in a nasal smear can give additional information about allergy, although there are a lot of false positives and negatives. Symptoms can be induced by application of the allergen to the nasal mucosa, which results in an immediate and late-phase reaction (three to ten hours) after the provocation (Figure 11-2).

The exact pathophysiological mechanism will be detailed elsewhere; briefly, however, the allergen binds to two neighboring IgE antibodies, fixed to the membrane of a mast cell or basophil. Allergic mediators such as histamine, serotonin, and sulfidopeptidoleukotrienes: a mixture of LTC_4, LTD_4, and LTE_2, which are lipoxygenase products of arachidonic acid, eosinophil-chemotactic factor, and tryptase are released by these cells during both the reactions. Prostaglandins, cycloexygenase products of arachidonic acid, are also released and with leukotrienes cause inflammatory reactions. Prostaglandin D_2, exclusively derived from

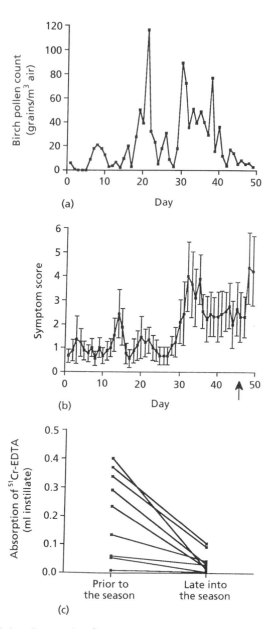

Figure 11-1. Composite figure showing daily birch pollen counts (a), daily symptom scores (b), and absorption of a radioactive tracer (c). Reproduced with permission from Grieff L, Wollmer P, Svensson C, et al. Effect of seasonal allergic rhinitis on airway mucosal absorption of chromium-S1-labelled EDTA. Thorax 1993;48:648–650.

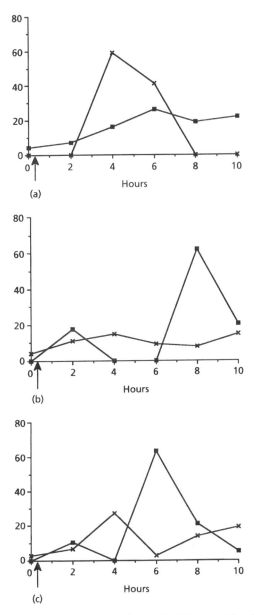

Figure 11-2. Three representative individuals with the relative changes in methacholine-induced nasal secretion and the total number of eosinophils prior to and every second hour up to 10 hours after a nasal allergen challenge. ■, Percentage changes in the total number of eosinophils; X, percentage changes in methacholine-induced nasal secretions. The arrows indicate the nasal allergen challenge (10,000 biological units). Reprinted from Busse WW, Holgate ST. Asthma and Rhinitis. Boston: Blackwell Science, 1995.

mast cells, is the only mediator that does not appear in the late reaction, which suggests that mast cells are not involved. The allergen-induced late-phase reaction is marked by an early influx of eosinophils, and later basophils and neutrophils.

The production of IgE is regulated by the lymphocytes and more specifically by a fine interaction between T-helper and T-suppressor cells. Interleukins play a major role in the activity of and interaction between lymphocytes.

Noninfectious nonallergic rhinitis

Vasomotor rhinitis: In the mucosa of the nose, the smooth muscles of arterioles and venules are innervated by the autonomic nervous system. Sympathetic stimulation results in vasoconstriction, while parasympathetic stimulation causes congestion. The most important result of parasympathetic action, however, is secretion by the nasal glands. One of the causes of vasomotor rhinopathy, which is a more correct term, may be an imbalance of the autonomic nervous system in favor of the parasympathetic system. This pathogenetic mechanism explains the predominant complaints of rhinorrhea.

Neurotransmitters and neuropeptides, released in the autonomic nervous system, exert homeostatic control of nasal secretion and vascular tonus. Vasoactive intestinal polypeptide is demonstrated in parasympathetic nerve fibers. In the sensory pathways, calcitonin gene-related peptide, substance P, and neurokinin A participate in axon response-mediated vasodilatation. The pathophysiology of vasomotor rhinitis might involve an exaggeration of these neural influences.

Fairbanks lists a variety of factors that may interfere with the vasomotor system, such as temperature, humidity, recumbency, or lack of airflow in laryngectomy patients or choanal atresia. Irritation by chemicals, dust, or tobacco smoke can also elicit a vasomotor reaction. Drugs can cause rhinopathy when they are applied topically or systemically. Mucosal swelling may be the result of acetylsalicylic acid, oral contraceptives, hydantoin, rauwolfia preparations, etc. Dryness of the mucosa is caused by atropine, corticosteroids, or catecholamine derivatives. A well-known example of the latter is the abuse of decongestant nose drops. Hypothyroidism, emotional causes, and pregnancy or premenstrual colds are examples of hormonally induced vasomotor rhinopathy. Estrogens cause vascular engorgement not only in the uterus but also in the nose. Furthermore, the nasal mucosa in pregnant women shows glandular hyperreactivity.

Eosinophilic rhinitis: Nonallergic rhinitis with eosinophilia syndrome (NARES) is a term introduced by Mullarkey et al. They found >20% eosinophils in the nasal smear of patients with sneezing attacks, watery rhinorrhea, itchy feeling, and incomplete obstruction without other demonstrable pathology. It is detected in 15% of rhinitis cases. Eosinophils have a proinflammatory function, and they inhibit the mediators of mast cells but also exert a cytotoxic effect. The syndrome has a familial history, and it usually starts during adulthood and is responsible for the majority of rhinitis in the aged. The two main criteria for NARES are 1) >20% eosinophils in nasal smear, and 2) no demonstrable allergy. In this subgroup of rhinitis, nasal polyps and asthma are frequent. When those signs and symptoms are absent in an early stage of the disease, patients often develop them later in life. It is suggested that NARES is the early phase of the triad. In that group of patients an increasing aspirin (ASA) intolerance is observed with age. Some authors consider NARES as a variant of vasomotor rhinitis and call it perennial intrinsic rhinitis. Wayoff et al think it is a link between vasomotor rhinitis and ASA-triad.

HYPERREACTIVITY

The concept of nasal hyperreactivity is derived from earlier studies on bronchial hyperreactivity. Commonly used stimuli were histamine and acetylcholine, which caused a dose-dependent relationship in asthmatic patients. However, it will be clear that nasal and bronchial hyperreactivity cannot be compared easily when taking the differences in the target organs into account.

Hyperreactivity or hyperresponsiveness of the nasal mucosa is an increased sensitivity to nonspecific stimuli or irritants. It can be described as a clinical feature of any kind of rhinitis. The nose exaggerates in its reaction to daily-life stimuli such as dust particles, temperature changes, smoke, and perfumes. Hyperreactivity can be a state of the nasal mucosa following an episode of infectious rhinitis. Patients may complain of nasal obstruction and nasal hypersecretion weeks or months after a viral or bacterial rhinitis or sinusitis, although there is not a single piece of evidence any more of an infection. Another example is the finding that patients with allergic rhinitis react in a more pronounced way to nonspecific stimuli, such as histamine, than patients without nasal allergy. This may explain the fact that infections in allergic patients usually evolve more easily to the chronic stages than infections in patients without allergy.

The exact mechanism of hyperreactivity is unknown. Some hypotheses are increased epithelial permeability, increased sensitivity of nerve endings, modulation of afferent impulses in the central nervous system, changed number or sensitivity of cell receptors, and mediator release. Gerth van Wijk concluded that nasal hyperreactivity is important, especially in allergic rhinitis and to a lesser degree in vasomotor rhinitis; it is unimportant in infectious rhinitis. A biochemically or clinically defined late-phase reaction did not necessarily accompany a change in hyperreactivity. The author concluded that the cellular influx observed during the late nasal reaction is not a prerequisite for the induction of nasal hyperreactivity.

RHINITIS AS PART OF A SYSTEMIC DISEASE
Mucociliary dysfunction: ciliary dyskinesis

The dynein arms that contain ATP-ase transform chemical energy into mechanical energy. When dynein is missing, the action of sliding microtubules becomes defective, which results in an absent mucociliary transport system and immobile spermatozoa. In 1933, Kartagener described a syndrome with the triad of bronchiectasis, chronic sinusitis, and situs inversus.

The term "primary ciliary dyskinesia" is preferred rather than "immotile cilia syndrome," since one third of all ciliated cells have mobile cilia, although in an abnormal pattern. Ciliary beat frequency is an important parameter, but the coordination of the various cilia contributes to an effective mucociliary clearance. Symptoms of dyskinetic cilia are chronic sinusitis, bronchiectasis, situs inversus (Kartagener's syndrome) but also rhinitis, nasal polyposis, chronic and recurrent otitis media, male infertility, and absent or underdeveloped frontal sinuses. "Primary" means that it has a genetic origin. The mode of inheritance is autosomal recessive. The gene for the presence (or absence) of ciliary mobility probably controls the situs of the viscera during the embryogenesis. Absence of control allows situs to be determined in a random fashion, which explains the 50% of the patients shown to have Kartagener's syndrome.

In 1970, Young described a group of men presenting with infertility due to obstructive azoospermia; 54% of the 52 patients had severe chest disease. The cause of the obstruction was not entirely clear. All studies of Young's syndrome describe normal ultrastructure of respiratory cilia and sperm. However, nasal cilia in brushings and biopsy were immotile or dyskinetic. Smallman supposed that there is a possible overlap between primary ciliary dyskinesia and Young's syndrome.

Ultrastructural changes are also found in cilia from patients with chronic sinusitis, nasal polyposis, rhinitis medicamentosa, allergic rhinitis, and cystic fibrosis. These changes are acquired, so they are called secondary. In these cases of secondary ciliary dyskinesia, microtubular abnormalities (9 + 3, 9 + 1, 9 + 4, 10 + 0, etc.), membrane abnormalities, intracellular inclusions, disorientation, and radial spoke defects have been demonstrated. It has been shown that up to 10% of cilia may be abnormal in patients with acquired respiratory conditions and up to 5% of cilia are structurally aberrant in normal children.

Cystic fibrosis

Cystic fibrosis (CF) is an autosomal recessive disorder of the exocrine glandular function. It is characterized by pancreatic insufficiency with malabsorption, salt wasting, and dehydration. The diagnosis can be made by a sweat test. The pulmonary lesions are progressive due to a thick sticky mucus which results in either complete or partial obstruction of the bronchioles. Nasal polyposis and sinusitis occur in 10% and 11% of patients, respectively. In the past, a ciliary dyskinesia factor in the serum was thought to be responsible for the defective mucociliary transport, but this suggestion has been withdrawn. The transport is rather inhibited by the thick layer of mucus that interferes with the ciliary movements.

Sarcoidosis

In sarcoidosis, characteristic submucosal yellow nodules appear. Probably they are granulomes and consist of epithelial cells with multinucleated giant cells but without caseation. Other clinical symptoms are mucosal dryness with crusting and obstruction by mass. Sarcoidosis is suspected when nasal symptoms are combined with cervical or hilar adenopathy, chronic pulmonary findings and infiltrates on chest radiographs, skin lesions, and increased ACE or calcium serum level. The etiology is unknown, but there is a depression of the delayed type hypersensitivity. The Kveim test is often positive.

Connective tissue disorders

The nasal mucosa can be affected as a manifestation of a systemic disease. Connective tissue disorders may have vasculitis as their hallmark, others have granulomas, still others have both. There is evidence for systemic lupus erythematosus, Sjögren's syndrome, or relapsing polychondritis being autoimmune diseases. Other connective tissue disorders are polyarteritis nodosa, which is characterized by necrotizing vasculitis; Behçet's disease, which may be called an autoimmune disease with aphtous ulcerations of the upper aerodigestive tract and genitalia; and Churg-Strauss syndrome, which consists of a triad of systemic vasculitis, asthma, and tissue eosinophilia with polyps as the nasal finding. Sometimes the vasculitis and mucosal ulcerations result in septal perforation and nasal saddling.

Hematopoietic dysfunction

Nasal findings in hematopoietic disorders such as acute lymphoblastic leukemia and anaplastic leukemia are petechial and ulcerative lesions of the nasal mucosa. In non-Hodgkin's lymphoma, extranodal manifestations like mucosal gums can occur, which can be destructive to the nasal skeleton.

Diseases affecting the midface

Midline destructive disorders, so-called "midline granulomas," comprise a variety of diseases that present as destructive lesions in the upper airways. They include infectious, immune, and neoplastic disorders. A chronic and destructive ulcerative lesion of the midface can be caused by leishmaniasis. The etiology of Wegener's granulomatosis is unknown. It is a granulomatous disease with marked predilection for the respiratory tract. The granulomas have central necrosis, a stellate morphology, and an outer ring of pallisading histiocytes. Other manifestations are systemic vasculitis and focal necrotising glomerulonephritis. Concerning the nose, there is increasing nasal obstruction with serosanguineous rhinorrhea and crusts. Septal perforation and saddling are common features. Diagnosis is made by determining antineutrophil cytoplasm antibodies (ANCA) that are increased. Patients often suffer from anemia. Blood tests further show elevated sedimentation rate and abnormal urine sediment.

Lethal midline granuloma is also a clinical term used for a nonspecific destructive midfacial lesion. It is strongly related to a malignant lymphoma with T-cell identity. In that case it is closely associated with an infection with the Epstein-Barr virus.

SELECTED REFERENCES

Anggard A, Lundberg JM, Lundblad L. Nasal autonomic innervation with special reference to peptidergic nerves. Eur J Respir Dis 1983;64(suppl 128):143–148.

Binford CH, Meyers WM, Walsh GP. Leprosy. JAMA 1982;247: 2283–2292.

Cepero R, Smith RJ, Catlin FI, et al. Cystic fibrosis—an otolaryngologic perspective. Otolaryngol Head Neck Surg 1987;97:356–360.

Corey JP, Romberger CP, Shaw GY. Fungal diseases of the sinuses. Otolaryngol Head Neck Surg 1990;103:1012–1015.

Dieges PH, Wentges RThR. Allergische rhinopathie. Amsterdam: Mondeel, 1979.

Fairbanks DNF. Non allergic rhinitis. In: Cummings CW, Fredrickson JM, Harker LA, et al., eds. Otolaryngology—head and neck surgery. St. Louis: C.V. Mosby, 1986:663–672.

Gerth van Wijk R. Nasal hyperreactivity. Thesis. Erasmus University, Rotterdam, 1991.

Gwaltney JM, Hayden FG. The nose and infection. In: Proctor DF, Andersen I, eds. The nose. Amsterdam: Elsevier, 1982.

Hill JH. Infections. In: Cummings CW, Fredrickson JM, Harker LA, et al., eds. Otolaryngology—head and neck surgery. St. Louis: C.V. Mosby, 1986:585–595.

Holinger PH, Gelman HK, Wolfe CK. Rhinoscleroma of the lower respiratory tract. Laryngoscope 1977;87:1–9.

Johns CJ. Sarcoidosis. In: Isselbacher KJ, Adams RD, Braunwald E, et al., eds. Harrison's principles of internal medicine. Tokyo: Kosaido Printing Co., 1980:928–932.

Kartagener M. Zur pathogenese der bronchiektasien. I. Bronchiektasien bei situs viscerum inversus. Beitr Klin Tuberk 1933;83:489–509.

McDonald TJ. Manifestations of systemic disease. In: Cummings CW, Fredrickson JM, Harker LA, et al., eds. Otolaryngology—head and neck surgery. St. Louis: C.V. Mosby, 1986: 597–609.

Mullarkey MF, Hill JS, Webb R. Allergic and nonallergic rhinitis: their characterization with attention to the meaning of eosinophilia. J Allergy Clin Immunol 1980;65:122–126.

O'Connor JC, Robinson RA. Review of diseases presenting as "midline granuloma." Acta Otolaryngol (Stockh) 1987; 439(suppl):1–16.

Schatz M, Zeiger RS. Diagnosis and management of rhinitis during pregnancy. Allergy Proc 1988;9:545–554.

Stockmann G. The status of Churg-Strauss syndrome among other hypereosinophilic granulomatous and vasculitis diseases. Z Rheumatol 1988;47:388–396.

Van Cauwenberge P. Epidemiology of the common cold. Rhinology 1985;23:273–282.

Van Cauwenberge P. Micro-organisms involved in nasal and sinusal infections. Rhinology 1981;19(suppl):29–40.

Waldman SR et al. Nasal tuberculosis: a forgotten entity. Laryngoscope 1981;91:11–16.

Wayoff M, Moneret-Vautrin DA, Hsieh V. The nonallergic rhinitis with eosinophils. In: Passali D, ed. Around the nose. Florence: Conti Tipocolor, 1988:101–110.

Young D. Surgical treatment of male infertility. J Reprod Fertil 1970;23:541–542.

Pathophysiology of Allergic and Nonallergic Rhinitis

12

INTRODUCTION

Allergic rhinitis is the most common form of allergic disease and afflicts about 10 to 20% of the general population, although the incidence may be increasing. Allergic rhinitis can be divided into seasonal and perennial types. Seasonal allergic rhinitis is often called hay fever in the fall or rose fever in the spring and is due to pollen exposure. Perennial rhinitis has triggering allergens such as house dust mite, animal dander, and mold allergens. Introduction of techniques for in vivo harvesting of nasal surface fluid and the assays for biochemical markers, mediators, cytokines, cell surface proteins, gene expressions, and extracellular matrix molecules has advanced our knowledge of the pathophysiology and pharmacology of allergic rhinitis. Although the symptoms of allergic and nonallergic rhinitis are similar, the pathophysiological events leading to the nasal symptoms may be quite different. In the present chapter, the main focus will be on the recent increased knowledge of the pathophysiology of allergic rhinitis.

ANATOMY

Squamous epithelium covers the anterior part of the nose, whereas ciliated pseudostratified epithelium blankets the remaining part of the nasal cavity. Pseudostratified epithelium consists of at least four cell types: ciliated columnar cells, nonciliated columnar cells, goblet cells, and basal cells. Epithelial cells rest on a basement membrane with apical lateral portions connected by tight junctions. Goblet cells, serous glands, and seromucous glands contribute to the production of airway secretions covering the mucosal surface. Further sources of fluid are plasma solutes from mucosal exudation processes and condensed water recovered from exhaled air.

Nasal mucosa is innervated by sympathetic, parasympathetic, and sensory nerves. Sensory nerves run in the trigeminal nerve, and stimulation of sensory c-fibers results in symptoms of itching and sneezing. Histamine-induced itching and sneezing can be abolished by topical treatment with H_1 receptor antagonists, but not with H_2 antagonists. Neuropeptides in the nose are found in nerve fibers (substance P and calcitonin gene-related peptide) in the human nasal mucosa, neuropeptide Y in the sympathetic stellate ganglion and vasoactive intestinal peptide in the parasympathetic nerve fibers.

Human nasal mucosa has a highly developed capillary network with a subepithelial fenestrated layer of capillaries. Cavernous sinusoids are situated in the deepest parts of the lamina propria, regulating the blood content of the mucosa. In the lower part of the lamina propria there are arteriovenous shunts, which allow the blood to pass by the capillary network. It has been suggested that these shunts are involved in the thermoregulation of the nose. Normal exchange of solutes occurs across the capillary endothelium, whereas in inflammation the endothelium of the postcapillary venules regulates the plasma exudation process.

The nasal mucosa shows striking similarities in structural and functional aspects to the tracheobronchial mucosa. The respiratory epithelium with the basement membrane and the adjacent submucosa with microvessels and glands have the same appearance in both locations. The venous sinusoids, which are very abundant in the nose, have also recently been demonstrated in the bronchi.

THE ALLERGIC REACTION

In allergic rhinitis, when the mucosa is exposed to an allergen, the allergenic protein first gains access to the airway epithelium and then is processed by cells capable of presenting these proteins to immunocompetent cells. This leads to an increased production of immunoglobulins, specifically IgE. IgE antibodies bind primarily with the Fc portion to high-affinity receptors on mast cells and basophils and to low-affinity receptors on other cells, such as monocytes, eosinophils, and platelets (Figure 12-1). With allergen re-exposure, cross-bridging of two or more IgE molecules on the surface of the cells results in production and release of biochemical mediators and other biological substances such as cytokines. Released substances act on the local cells and sensory nerve endings, leading to an increased blockage of the nose, watery and proteinic discharge, sneezes, and nasal itching. These symptoms characterize the early allergic reaction.

Following the immediate allergic reaction, a continuous influx of inflammatory cells occurs in the nasal mucosal surface with resulting increased reactivity of the nose ("priming") to both allergenic and nonallergenic stimuli. In some patients, a single allergen provocation after some hours also leads to renewed symptoms and a second round of mediator release (late-phase response) with a recurrence of symptoms. Natural pollen exposure is probably a more complicated event in that there is an escalating mixture of the immediate, priming, nasal late-phase response, and an increased reactivity to nonspecific stimuli.

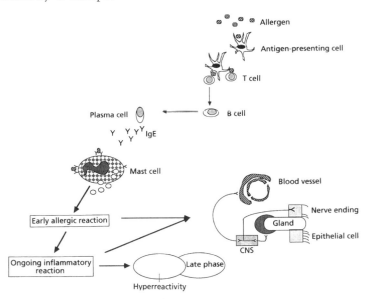

Figure 12-1. A schematic figure outlining the course of events leading to the immediate allergic reaction and the ongoing inflammatory response, which is characterized by an increased reactivity and a nasal late-phase response. CNS: Central nervous system. Reprinted from Busse WW, Holgate ST. Asthma and Rhinitis. Boston: Blackwell Science, 1995.

CELLULAR ASPECTS

Mast cells and basophils

Crucial cells in the allergic reaction are the mast cell and the basophil. These cells are distinguished by their basophil and metachromatic cytoplasmic granulae. Activation of the metha-chromatic cells is triggered by allergen-IgE binding which leads to release of preformed mediators from the granulae and a de novo synthesis of mediators from the mast cell membrane as well as a transcription and synthesis of cytokines.

During natural pollen exposure, the mast cells in the nasal mucosa are redistributed from their normal preseasonal habitat in the stroma into the epithelium, a finding which has been inter-preted as an intraepithelial migration of mucosal mast cells. In contrast, the blood basophil and its migratory capacity are contro-versial during natural pollen exposure.

Following allergen challenge, increased levels of mediators with specific mast cell origin such as tryptase and prostaglandin D_2 have been seen, as well as histamine and sulfidopeptido-leukotrienes (Figure 12-2). Histamine is still the only mediator that, locally applied, mimics the nasal symptoms of the early allergic nasal reaction. Histamine acts through binding to receptors on the endothelial cells, vascular smooth muscles, and sensory nerves lead-

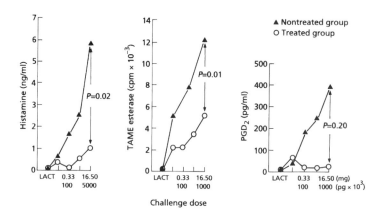

Figure 12-2.   Nasal challenge model: ragweed pollen, showing the mean change in mediator levels. Reproduced with permission from Creticos PS, Adkinson Jr NF, Kagey-Sobotka A, et al. Nasal challenge with ragweed pollen in hay fever patients. J Clin Invest 1985;76: 2247–2253.

ing to plasma exudation, vasodilatation, and secretion, respectively. Histamine also induces a reflex-mediated parasympathetic glandular secretion. The tissue levels of histamine correlated with the patient's nasal symptoms during the pollen season. High levels of free histamine are commonly seen in the unchallenged nasal cavity.

The importance of histamine as a mediator is clearly supported by the beneficial effect of antihistamines on symptoms during natural disease and on symptoms and mediator release in the challenge situation. Histamine, however, cannot attract and activate eosinophils. Histamine also cannot induce an increased reactivity of the nasal mucosa to specific or nonspecific stimuli, nor can it produce late-phase reactions after single challenges. These aspects do not exclude the possibility that histamine is associated with both the immediate and late-phase allergic reactions.

Pathophysiology of the reappearance of nasal symptoms after an allergen challenge is not fully elucidated. These late nasal symptoms may be linked to an influx of cells or to a second round of mediator release or plasma exudation. A similar pattern of mediator release as seen with the early response is seen in some individuals observed over hours after the initial allergen challenge. Alternatively, early influx and activation of inflammatory cells into the nasal secretions after allergen challenge has been seen within one hour, much earlier than any late-phase reactions. Furthermore, the inflammatory cell influx was not followed by any obvious nasal symptoms in most patients. The inflammatory cell influx alone may not be a helpful index of the late-phase response to allergen.

The eosinophil

This cell has been associated with allergic disease in that a direct relationship between the influx of eosinophils into the nasal mucosa and allergic rhinitis is noted. In contrast, eosinophils are absent from the nasal secretions during asymptomatic periods. Eosinophils can produce and release several biological substances. Enzymes are capable of degrading mast cell products such as histamine, leukotrienes, and cytotoxic proteins such as major basic protein (MBP), eosinophil peroxidase (EPO), eosinophil cationic protein (ECP), and eosinophil protein X (EPX). Desquamation and denudation of the airway epithelium during eosinophilic inflammation would expose underlying nerve endings and provide an attractive explanation for the induction of airway hyperreactivity. Increased numbers of eosinophils in association with late lower-airway responses have been a source of support for the hypothesis associating a link between airway hyperresponsiveness and the influx and activation of eosinophils.

Nasal provocation experiments fail to demonstrate a simple link between eosinophils and increased airway responsiveness to methacholine. An early rise in eosinophil number on the nasal mucosal surface occurs after allergen challenge, and the secretory responsiveness to methacholine is increased. However, no clear relationship between these two events was demonstrated. Some patients showed a very rapid increase in eosinophil number and a slower increase in secretory responsiveness, or vice versa. Antihistamines abolish the allergen-induced increase in nasal secretory responsiveness to methacholine without reducing the number of eosinophils on the mucosal surface. Finally, morphological changes such as a loss of the epithelial lining and a disruption of epithelial integrity have not been found in the nasal mucosa in biopsies taken during naturally occurring rhinitis or directly after a nasal allergen challenge. Complement fragments, cytokines, and other factors may possess eosinophil chemotactic capacity. Platelet-activating factor (PAF) delivered topically produces a rapid and transient increase in the number of eosinophils on the nasal mucosal surface in allergic subjects. Yet influx of eosinophils was not associated with any increased nasal reactivity.

Neutrophils

The neutrophil is more often associated with infectious disease because of its phagocytotic capacity. The number of neutrophils increases on the mucosal surface hours after a nasal allergen challenge. Neutrophils contain and release hydrolases, proteases, myeloperoxidases (MPO), and other enzymes. As a marker of neutrophil activation, the levels of MPO increased in nasal lavage fluid during seasonal exposure to pollen allergen, suggesting neutrophil activation during the inflammatory process. There were no correlations between the patient's symptoms and the levels of MPO. In vitro findings suggest that the neutrophil can produce arachidonic metabolites such as 5-HETE, LTB_4, and PGE_2.

Antigen presenting cells (APC)

The immune system possesses the capacity to recognize allergenic proteins when these molecules gain access to the mucosa. In atopy, the classic example is the induction of β-lymphocytes to produce IgE antibodies. All cells which express class II MHC (Ia) on their surface, such as dendritic cells, monocytes/macrophages, β-lymphocytes, and epithelial cells, could exert antigen presenting properties for T-lymphocytes. Both macrophages and Langerhans cells have been found to reside in the nasal mucosa and in the submucosa. Furthermore, the number of macrophages increased on the mucosal surface after allergen challenge and also during seasonal exposure to allergen. Topical glucocorticoid treatment does not seem to alter the number of macrophages during natural pollinosis. The number of macrophages was further not related to the patient's symptoms during natural pollinosis. In similarity, the number of CD1$^+$ cells, presumably Langerhans cells, increased in the nasal mucosa during the pollen season and very early after allergen challenge. Topical glucocorticoid treatment reduced the number of Langerhans cells.

Lymphocytes

T cells can functionally be divided into two distinct populations, helper T cells and cytolytic T cells. In response to antigen stimulation, helper T cells can secrete cytokines, whose function is to promote the proliferation and differentiation of T cells and other cells. Functionally distinct populations of T cells express different membrane proteins, which serve as phenotypic markers of different lymphocyte populations. Most helper T cells express a surface protein called CD4$^+$, and most cytotoxic T cells express a different marker called CD8$^+$. Antibodies against such markers can be used to identify various lymphocyte populations.

Little attention has been paid to the potential role and presence of lymphocytes in the nasal mucosa. Recently, biopsies from allergic patients and nonallergic controls failed to show any difference between the number of helper T cells and cytotoxic T cells in the epithelium. However, in the lamina propria, a higher number of activated CD$^+$ T cells was expressed in the allergic group. Following a local allergen challenge of the nose, increased numbers of CD4$^+$ helper T cells and CD25$^+$ cells, presumed T lymphocytes, have been found in the nasal submucosa. It seems that allergen could promote T-cell activation and proliferation, thereby augmenting and sustaining the allergic reaction.

Nasal epithelium

The nasal epithelium is an important barrier, also valuable for transport and secretory functions. Based on in vitro studies, the epithelium could participate in antigen presentation through antigen-binding surface proteins. The ability of the epithelium to generate mediators and cytokines suggests an active involvement in the inflammatory process. The epithelial cells may play an important role for the local recruitment, differentiation, and survival of inflammatory migrating cells.

An increased absorption of allergens and other foreign materials is a feature of allergic rhinitis and asthma. This hypothesis has been attractive although the results supporting it are weak. Provocation with an inflammatory stimulus such as histamine results in a prompt exudative response with unfiltered plasma leakage across the airway endothelial–epithelial barriers onto the airway lumen. The dramatic increase in outward exudative permeability, however, is not accompanied by any changes of the inward absorption permeability as measured by absorption of radioactive tracers in direct contact with the nasal mucosa for 15 minutes during the exudative response. In seasonal allergic rhinitis, the inward absorption permeability is unchanged or even decreased.

ALLERGIC RHINITIS DURING NATURAL EXPOSURE

Investigators have shown a correlation between the tosyl-L-arginine-methyl-esterase activity in the daily recovered lavage fluids and the nasal symptoms as well as the number of birch pollen grains in the air. In seasonal allergic rhinitis, increased levels of both albumin and bradykinin in nasal lavage fluids have been demonstrated and reflect exudation of plasma proteins and activation of plasma protein systems with the formation of proinflammatory mediators. An increased number of eosinophils and raised levels of eosinophil cationic protein (ECP) on the nasal mucosal surface is also seen during natural allergic rhinitis. These changes were accompanied by an increased secretory responsiveness of the nasal mucosa to methacholine. This also could be demonstrated during a very mild pollen season that did not produce any significant increase in nasal symptoms. Both the increases in number and activation of eosinophils and the increased secretory responsiveness to methacholine were significantly inhibited by topical glucocorticoids.

In seasonal studies of birth pollen–induced rhinitis, the exposure to pollens has at the end of the season diminished. Yet patients had more pronounced symptoms and experienced more nasal complaints at the season endings. This finding suggests the presence of a naturally acquired hyperreactivity to allergen. Late into the pollen season, the absorption of a radioactive tracer (51-

Cr-EDTA) across the nasal mucosa was signifi᷅ some weeks prior to the season at a time-point ᴠ were asymptomatic. At the end of the birch-ᴘ increased exudative responsiveness to histamine wₑ pared to the same histamine dose at a symptom-ᴛ outside the season. Studies carried out during natuᵣ ᴏccurring allergic rhinitis have demonstrated an increased mucosal exudation of plasma, secretory hyperreactivity, an increased number and activation of both mast cells and eosinophils, and a reduced absorption permeability.

PHARMACOLOGICAL TREATMENT

The efficacy of glucocorticoids has given new and important information concerning the pathophysiology of allergic rhinitis. Almost all inflammatory cell types are affected by glucocorticoids. In nasal challenge experiments, oral steroids given 48 hours prior to allergen challenge effectively reduce the increase in later-occurring nasal symptoms and associated release of mediators. Topical glucocorticoids initiated after an initial allergen challenge and continued up to allergen rechallenge 24 hours later inhibit the increased nasal symptoms and the increased levels of TAME-esterase activity in the nasal lavage fluid. A longer pretreatment time (one week) reduces both the allergen-induced increase to renewed allergen challenge and the allergen-induced increase in histamine-induced nasal reactivity. Plasma exudation, which is considered a reflection of the inflammatory condition of the nasal mucosa, and the generation of plasma-derived mediators are also effectively reduced by topical glucocorticoid treatment during native disease.

New nonsedating antihistamines also possess properties that may not be directly related to a H_1-receptor antagonism. This includes finding a reduction of allergen-induced histamine and TAME-esterase release into the nasal cavity. These results, in conjunction with observations that these drugs in nasal challenge procedures reduced the allergen-induced secretory responsiveness, have raised the question of whether the clinical beneficial effects of antihistamines may also to some extent be related to pharmacological properties not directly related to a blocking of the H_1-receptors.

Topical cromolyn is an effective treatment in alleviating nasal symptoms during seasonal allergic rhinitis, but less effective than glucocorticoids. Nedocromil sodium has been found to inhibit ergen-induced mast cell mediator release in vitro and in vivo and to inhibit the infiltration of mast cells into the nasal mucosa during seasonal exposure to allergen.

NONALLERGIC RHINITIS

A common estimate of the prevalence of nonallergic rhinitis has been about 5 to 10% in the general population. However, a questionnaire distributed in Sweden has estimated >20% of patients suffering from nonallergic complaints with a duration of more than six months. Yet only 2 to 4% suffer from symptoms demanding medical treatment. The diagnosis of nonallergic rhinitis is based on exclusion, where allergy by standard routine procedures cannot be determined.

Nonallergic rhinitis is characterized by the presentation of nasal symptoms on exposure to everyday life stimuli such as chemical irritants, tobacco smoke, perfumes, cold air, food, red wine, spices, or sexual excitement. Many individuals can show nasal symptoms on exposure to some of the above-mentioned stimuli but do not report their symptoms as nasal complaints. This overlap probably also reflects the fact that there is no uniformly accepted definition of nonallergic rhinitis.

Pathophysiology

The absorption permeability of the nasal mucosa in specific subgroups of nonallergic rhinitic patients remains to be examined. Other explanations of the pathophysiology include factors such as an increased sensitivity of glandular cholinoceptors or a hypersensitivity of the irritant sensory receptors. It has also been speculated that a changed modulation of the afferent impulses in the central nervous system could explain this feature.

A model has been set up to challenge nonallergic rhinitic patients by the use of cold dry air. By performing nasal lavages after the cold dry air challenges, Togias et al have found release of histamine and prostaglandin D_2, among other mediators, into the nasal lavage fluid which suggests mast cell activation. Furthermore, a later recurrence of nasal symptoms is associated with increased levels of histamine and TAME-esterase activity in the recovered lavage fluid. Cold dry air challenge resembles allergen challenge to sensitized subjects, yet by contrast to allergen challenge, a tricyclic antihistamine could not inhibit symptoms or histamine release after cold dry air challenge. Whether mediator release also occurs during the natural exposure to cold air in these patients is unknown. It is not yet known whether the mediator release is due to the low temperature or the dryness of the air.

Other ways of stimulating the nose include the ingestion of hot, spicy food such as hot chili pepper. The food-induced nasal rhinorrhea is blocked by pretreatment with atropine. The hot chili pepper contains capsaicin, which produces a similar secretory response when applied topically to the nasal and oral mucosa. Neurogenic stimuli, nicotine applied on the nasal mucosa, induces glandular secretion, noted by a dose-dependent rise in fucose levels. Nicotine, however, does not induce any plasma exudate response. Thus neurogenic inflammation does not seem to be a feature of the human upper airways.

SUMMARY

Allergic inflammatory airway conditions are increasingly common. Recent decades have witnessed rapidly increasing information about the pathophysiology, pharmacology, and cell biology of these conditions. The accessibility of the human nasal mucosa provides flexibility for studies of inflammatory airway diseases. The result of such studies not only may serve the purpose of revealing the nasal inflammatory process but may also indicate which pathophysiological events may occur in the tracheobronchial airways. Seasonal allergic rhinitis is now subject to extensive investigations in laboratory challenge experiments and more importantly under natural disease conditions. Perennial allergic rhinitis and different forms of nonallergic rhinitis now remain largely unexplored in terms of mucosal mechanisms and abnormalities. Studies of the latter conditions with novel nasal techniques hold great promise for new important insights into the pathophysiology and pharmacology of airway diseases.

SELECTED REFERENCES

Andersson M, Andersson P, Pipkorn U. Topical glucocorticosteroids and allergen-induced increase in nasal reactivity; relationship between treatment time and inhibitory effect. J Allergy Clin Immunol 1988;82:1019–1026.

Andersson M, Svensson C, Andersson P, Pipkorn U. Objective monitoring of the allergic inflammatory response of the nasal mucosa in hayfever patients during natural allergen exposure.

Am Rev Respir Dis 1989;139:911–914.

Ballow M. Lymphocytes, monocytes, macrophages and neutrophils. J Allergy Clin Immunol 1989;84:1019–1023.

Cauna N, Hinderer KH. Fine structure of blood vessels of the human nasal respiratory mucosa. Ann Otol Rhinol Laryngol 1969;78:865–879.

Chandra RK, Heresi G, Woodford G. Double-blind, controlled crossover trial of 4% intranasal sodium chromoglycate solution in patients with seasonal allergic rhinitis. Ann Allergy 1982;49:131–134.

Cox G, Ohtoshi T, Vancheri C, et al. Promotion of eosinophil survival by human bronchial epithelial cells and its modulation by steroids. Am J Respir Cell Mol Biol 1991;4:525–531.

Enerback L, Pipkorn U, Granerus G. Intraepithelial migration of nasal mucosal mast cells in hay fever. Int Arch Allergy Immunol 1986;80:44–51.

Eyermann C. Nasal manifestations of allergy. Ann Otol Rhinol Laryngol 1927;36:808–815.

Fokkens WJ, Vroom TM, Rijntes E, Mulder PGH. Fluctuation of the number of CD1 (T6), HLA-DR expressing cells, presumably Langerhans cells, in the nasal mucosa of patients with an isolated grass-pollen allergy before, during and after the grass pollen season. J Allergy Clin Immunol 1989;84:39–43.

Jessen M, Janzon L. Prevalence of non-allergic nasal complaints in an urban and a rural population in Sweden. Allergy 1989;44:582–587.

Holm AF, Fokkens WJ, Godthelp T, et al. Effect of 3 months' nasal steroid therapy on nasal T cells and Langerhans cells in patients suffering from allergic rhinitis. Allergy 1995;50:204–209.

Mygind N. Perennial rhinitis. In: Mygind N, ed. Essential allergy. N. Blackwell Scientific Publications, 1986:313.

Mygind N, Borum P. Nasal provocation tests. In: Kerr JW, Ganderton MA, eds. Proc XI Int Congress of Allergol Clin Immunol. London: Macmillan, 1983:207–212.

Perki JM. Allergy in general practice. Practitioner 1972;208:776–783.

Pipkorn U, Proud D, Schleimer RP, et al. Effect of short term systemic glucocorticoid treatment on human nasal mediator release after antigen challenge. J Clin Invest 1987;80:957–961.

Shaw RJ, Fitzharris P, Cromwell O, et al. Allergen-induced release of sulphopeptide leukotrienes (SRS-A) and LTB4 in allergic rhinitis. Allergy 1985;40:1–6.

Svensson C. Exudation of plasma into human airways. On the regulation of exudative responses in human nasal mucosa. Thesis. Lund: University Hospital, 199:1–164.

Tada T, Ishizaka K. Distribution of gamma E-forming cells in lymphoid tissues of the human and monkey. J Immunol 1970;104:377–387.

Uddman R, Sundler F. Vasoactive intestinal polypeptide nerves in human upper respiratory tract. ORL 1979;41:221–226.

Wihl JA, Petersen N, Petersen LN, et al. Effect of the nonsedative H₁-receptor antagonist astemizole in perennial allergic and nonallergic rhinitis. J Allergy Clin Immunol 1985;75:720–727.

Nasal Polyposis

13

INTRODUCTION

Nasal polyps were first described more than 3000 years ago. This condition represents the most common group of mass lesions in the nose. In spite of the illustrious attention that nasal polyps have long received, there are many unresolved questions with respect to their pathogenesis. Nasal polyps represent a considerable management challenge. A testimony to this is the high rate of recurrence after polypectomy, 40 to 50%, still seen today. Nasal polyposis is in many respects a paradigm of chronic inflammation of the airways, and a substantial number of features are similar to those described in allergic rhinitis and asthma. Because of their location and gross anatomy, nasal polyps provide easy, even repeated, access to abundant human tissue for research purposes.

DEFINITION AND DESCRIPTIVE FEATURES

Nasal polyposis is a disease characterized by the presence of a hyperplastic, swollen, bulging mucosa in the nasal cavity that causes nasal obstruction. A nasal polyp appears as a smooth, pale mass with a pedunculated base. They are often multiple and most commonly arise from the mucosa of the paranasal sinuses, particularly the ethmoid sinuses. However, polyp tissue may project posteriorly through the choanal area and extend into the anterior portion of the nasopharynx. These antrochoanal polyps are commonly unilateral, occur most often in children and young adults, and are thought to represent 4 to 6% of all nasal polyps.

Nasal polyps often develop in subjects with a history of chronic rhinitis or pansinusitis. There is also a high incidence of asthma. Indeed, coexisting asthma has been reported in up to 72% of cases, but it is generally considered to have increased prevalence in patients with nasal polyps. Furthermore, patients with nasal polyps often have increased methacholine airway responsiveness even in the absence of clinical asthma. The association of asthma, nasal polyps, and ASA (acetyl-methyl-esterase) intolerance has been long recognized and it is often referred to as the "asthma triad." Allergy has been considered to be an important component of the pathogenesis of nasal polyposis for many years, but it is now clear that there is not an increased prevalence of atopy, or of allergic disorders, in patients with nasal polyps compared to the general population. There are no significant differences in the number of epithelial mast cells in nasal polyps from allergic and nonallergic subjects. Moreover, there are no statistically significant correlations between the density of eosinophils in the polyp tissue with either skin test reactivity or IgE serum concentration.

In addition to asthma, nasal polyps have been described in association with cystic fibrosis (CF) and with Kartagener's syndrome. The incidence of nasal polyps in CF is between 20 and 30%, and these patients do not have an increased prevalence of allergy compared to the general population. Therefore, nasal polyps appear to develop in individuals in whom there is widespread airway mucosal disease. Perhaps local mechanical factors at particular locations in the nasal cavity interact with the inflamed mucosa to lead to the formation of the polyp structure.

HISTOPATHOLOGY

The histologic appearance of nasal polyps is quite variable, from mostly edematous polyps at one end of the spectrum to mostly fibrotic polyps at the other end. It is unclear whether this variability represents truly distinct types of polyps or different stages in the natural history of polyp formation. Either way, the general histologic appearance of nasal polyps is one of inflammation with varying degrees of abnormalities in the tissue structure (i.e., in the epithelial and stromal compartments of the polyp).

Epithelial damage, either ulceration or desquamation, is frequently observed in nasal polyps, although it is not unusual to observe epithelial metaplasia interspersed between areas of marked erosion of the epithelium. A general, prominent feature of nasal polyps is the presence of a thickened basement membrane. Underneath the basement membrane, much of the polyp stroma appears edematous and contains an abundant amorphous substance, coarse fibrous material with the appearance of fibrin and obvious collagen bundles. Nasal polyps contain a rather striking density of long spindle-shape cells that stain positive with an anti-α smooth muscle actin antibody. The emergence of these myofibroblast-like cells, probably through differentiation of fibroblasts, has been documented in situations of chronic inflammation, as in asthma and pulmonary fibrosis, and may represent a more synthetically active type of fibroblast. Finally, in general no nerves can be seen in the polyp of the stroma, but some nerve fibers may be observed in the pedicles of some polyps.

A prominent feature of nasal polyps is inflammation involving inflammatory cells of a variety of cell types. Nasal polyps contain about twice the number of mast cells found in the normal respiratory mucosa, but this increase is allergy independent. Most mast cells in the epithelium are formalin sensitive, chloracetate esterase (CAE) negative, and chymase negative. In contrast, most mast cells in the stroma are formalin resistant, CAE positive, and, in general, positive for both chymase and tryptase. These differences in mast cell phenotype could be due to distinct microenvironmental factors. Lymphocytes are also observed in the polyp stroma, but there is no statistically significant difference in the density of lymphocytes between polyps and normal nasal mucosa. Nasal polyp tissues contain a very small number of activated lymphocytes as assessed by $CD25^+$ (IL-2 receptor) expression. Eosinophils are the most abundant inflammatory cell type and are present in the majority of nasal polyps. In non-CF polyps, the density of eosinophils is much greater than in control inferior turbinate tissues. In addition, three-quarters of eosinophils in the tissue are EG2 positive by immunohistochemistry, indicating that a majority of these cells are activated.

In nasal polyposis tissues from non-CF patients, almost three out of four cells in the tissue were structural cells and one in five cells in the tissue were eosinophils. There were four eosinophils for each lymphocyte.

Polyps occurring in patients with cystic fibrosis have some distinct characteristics. A general feature of these is the presence of an essentially normal basement membrane. Contrary to some traditional thoughts, the density and distribution of mucous glands in CF polyps is the same as in non-CF polyps. With respect to the inflammatory component of the polyp, eosinophils are rare and neutrophils are numerous in CF polyps, and few inflammatory cells are seen in the epithelial region.

PATHOGENESIS

The examination of nasal polyposis reveals that eosinophils are the most comparatively increased cell type. In addition, eosinophils represent by far the most prevalent inflammatory cell type and are present in the majority of tissues. Furthermore, a number of structural abnormalities in the nasal polyp tissue, particularly epithelial cell damage, can be mechanistically related to the presence of eosinophils or of eosinophil-derived products. While the precise mechanisms underlying polyp formation remain elusive, there is a strong positive correlation between the number of past polypectomies and the peripheral blood eosinophil count. Together, these data indicate that the mechanisms underlying the accumulation and activation of eosinophils in the nasal mucosa are probably of central importance to understanding nasal polyp development. These mechanisms are complex and involve, in all likelihood, a number of different cell types interacting with each other. Cytokines and growth factors are the means by which this multicellular communication is articulated. The following paragraphs discuss those molecules that have been identified on cells derived from nasal polyps or directly in the tissues.

Nasal fibroblasts and nasal epithelial cells produce granulocyte macrophage colony stimulating factor (GM–CSF) in vitro. Fibroblasts and epithelial cells derived from nasal polyposis tissues spontaneously release greater amounts of GM–CSF compared to cells isolated from the normal nasal mucosa. This suggests in vivo upregulation and indicates a possible role in the propagation of inflammation. A number of cells stained positive for GM–CSF, including monocytes, epithelial cells, and fibroblasts, but eosinophils were the most prevalent positive cell type. GM–CSF mRNA transcripts are observed almost exclusively on eosinophils, and approximately 25% of eosinophils in the nasal polyp tissues expressed positive GM–CSF signals. The eosinophil, which had to this point been regarded as a GM–CSF target, is in fact capable of being a source, perhaps major, of this cytokine.

Spontaneous survival of eosinophils isolated from nasal polyps in vitro is markedly prolonged compared to control peripheral blood eosinophils. This effect can be substantially abrogated by exposing the cells to either GM-CSF or GM-CSF receptor antibodies. IL-3 (Interleukin 3) and IL-5 have also been shown to enhance survival and induce activation of eosinophils. Whether these cytokines are also involved in regulatory autocrine loops in polyp eosinophils is not yet known.

Transforming growth factor 6 (TGF6) gene expression and immunohistochemical protein are localized in nasal polyp tissue but not in the normal nasal mucosa. In these tissues, expression of TGF6 was found almost exclusively in eosinophils. Regulation of extracellular matrix protein synthesis, stimulation of fibroblast proliferation, and modulation of the fibroblast phenotype are clearly significant effects of TGF6. TGF6 is an immunosuppressor and anti-inflammatory cytokine capable of inducing a broad spectrum of effects including inhibition of B and T cell proliferation, immunoglobulin secretion, generation of cytotoxicity, suppression of natural and lymphokine-activated killing by large granular lymphocytes, T lymphocyte adhesion to endothelium, and downregulation of macrophages. It is tempting to speculate that the relative lack of lymphocyte activity observed in nasal polyp tissues may in fact be the result of active suppression mediated by TGF6.

Platelet derived growth factor (PDGF) is an important growth and chemotactic factor first discovered as a granule-associated glycoprotein in platelets. The main role played by PDGF is that of a proliferation factor, particularly for fibroblasts and smooth muscle cells. PDGF-B has been found in nasal polyp tissue in situ hybridization. Almost half of the eosinophils infiltrating the tissue expressed PDGF-B transcripts, and there was a significant correlation between the proportion of eosinophils expressing TGF6 and PDGF-B in the tissues.

It is likely that other growth factors such as insulin growth factor (IGF) and epidermal growth factor (EGF), among others, participate in this fibroblastic/angioblastic response, eventually culminating in fibrosis. For example, IGF-1 is a well-known mitogen for both fibroblasts and epithelial cells. There is marked localization of IGF-1 in nasal polyp tissues. This was restricted almost exclusively to the polyp epithelium.

CONCLUDING HYPOTHESIS

Even though patients with nasal polyps have increased levels of peripheral blood eosinophils, nasal polyposis is a localized disease.

The mechanisms involved in the disregulation, namely perpetuation, of the inflammatory response and its consequences (fibrosis) must lie in the tissue itself. Two streams of data eventually converge and may provide some new insights into the pathogenesis of polyp development. One is the contribution of tissue structural cells, particularly fibroblasts and epithelial cells. Indeed, these cells may act as effector cells (i.e., are capable of producing a number of cytokines and growth factors with broad regulatory activities). The second concerns the eosinophil. Eosinophils not only are capable of producing a number of regulatory molecules but may in fact be a major source in the tissue. This suggests novel roles for the eosinophil with respect to not only the consequences, but also the regulation, of inflammation at mucosal sites.

These two streams of data may converge when one considers the question of how eosinophils may become upregulated active effectors. The initiating events in the formation of nasal polyps, especially in nonallergic people, remain unknown. Nevertheless, there are examples that indicate that short-lived airway mucosal injury can lead to chronic airway inflammation and disease. It is plausible that local injury caused by repeated exposure to allergen, in allergic subjects, or to unknown agents, in nonallergic subjects, could lead to activation of the tissue structural cells. This may set the stage for a tissue-driven response, to indicate that an upregulation in the effector phenotype of the tissue cells might determine the nature and consequences of the inflammatory response. The influx of peripheral blood eosinophils into a distinctively active tissue could very well lead, by induction or selection, to the emergence of autocrine/paracrine loops of stimulation in these cells. These mechanisms could play a major role to perpetuate localized tissue inflammation leading to tissue damage.

Diagnosis and treatment of nasal polyposis

Nasal polyposis is typically diagnosed by the characteristic appearance of the nasal tissue on examination. Nasal polyps are almost always bilateral. They may be minimal polyps high in the nasal cavity or grow to completely occlude the nostril. Unilateral masses in the nasal cavity may suggest benign or malignant tumors, and these should be evaluated by appropriate specialists when there is a question.

Typically, nasal polyps affect adults in the 30 to 60 age range, but may be observed earlier in life. The finding of nasal polyps in children under age 18 should alert the physician to the possibility

219

that the patient has cystic fibrosis. Sweat chloride testing to exclude this possibility should be considered.

Treatment of nasal polyps is not satisfactory. Since the disease is a chronic ongoing process, topical nasal corticosteroids are the mainstay of therapy (e.g., fluticasone two sprays every day or twice a day in each nostril). However, delivery of the topical nasal corticosteroid may be impaired by the presence of large obstructing polyps. In severe cases, a short-term course of oral corticosteroids (e.g., prednisone 10 to 15 mg three times a day for seven days, followed by 10 to 15 mg daily for seven days) may be useful. Patients who fail to respond to this treatment may need surgical polypectomy followed by long-term topical nasal corticosteroids. Efforts to control nasal polyps by medical approaches should be made since repeated polypectomies can result in atrophic rhinitis.

Patients with nasal polyps may be allergic to aeroallergens and have concomitant allergic rhinitis. As previously discussed, however, the pathogenesis of nasal polyps is not felt to be directly mediated by IgE antibodies. Antihistamines and anticholinergic topical nasal sprays (e.g., ipratroprium 0.03%) may be helpful in dealing with rhinorrhea, but neither will decrease the size of nasal polyps. Similarly, neither allergen avoidance nor allergen immunotherapy will affect nasal polyp formation.

Sensitivity to aspirin and other nonsteroidal anti-inflammatory drugs (NSAIDs) occurs frequently in patients with nasal polyps and can aggravate nasal symptoms in addition to provoking severe asthma in some individuals. Therefore, most patients are advised to avoid NSAIDs. Treating nasal polyps in aspirin-sensitive patients by desensitizing to aspirin has been attempted. This procedure has not gained widespread acceptance since there are risks of provoking severe reactions, and the long-term benefits are not clear.

Patients with nasal polyps are likely to have recurrent and chronic sinusitis since the polyp tissue obstructs the sinus ostia, particularly of the ethmoid and maxillary sinuses. Appropriate courses of antibiotics are useful, but recurrences are common because of the obstruction of the ostia, preventing drainage. Complete or limited computerized tomography (CT) scanning of the sinuses using coronal views can delineate the extent of sinusitis and visualize the osteomeatal units. Polypectomy, along with ethmoidectomy and functional endoscopic sinus surgery, can be beneficial in patients with persistent disease. Moreover, there is some data to suggest that aggressive treatment of nasal polyps with sinusitis may improve asthma symptoms in patients with difficult-to-control disease. Nonetheless, management of patients with recurrent sinusitis is difficult because polyp tissue tends to reform in spite of appropriate use of topical nasal corticosteroids, courses of oral steroids, and polypectomies.

SELECTED REFERENCES

Dolovich J, Ohtoshi T, Jordana M, et al. Nasal polyps: local inductive microenvironment in the pathogenesis of the inflammation. In: Mygind N, Pipkorn U, Dahl R, eds., Rhinitis and asthma. Similarities and differences. Copenhagen: Munksgaard, 1990:233–240.

Probst L, Stoney P, Jeney E, Hawke M. Nasal polyps, bronchial asthma and aspirin sensitivity. J Otolaryngol 1992;21:60–65.

Settipane GA. Nasal polyps. Immunol and Allergy Clinics of North America 1987;7:105–115.

Slavin RG. Allergy is not a significant cause of nasal polyps. Arch Otolaryngol Head Neck Surg 1992;118:343.

Stern RC, Boat TF, Wood RE, et al. Treatment and prognosis of nasal polyps in cystic fibrosis. Am J Dis Child 1982;136:1067–1070.

Allergic Rhinitis: Today's Approach to Treatment

14

INTRODUCTION

Therapy of allergic upper respiratory tract disease is based on several important concepts. The IgE-mediated allergic process is now recognized as the basis not only for the immediate symptoms (sneezing, itchy and watery eyes, rhinorrhea, and nasal congestion on exposure to a relevant allergen) but also for the late allergic phase with cellular influx perpetuating the clinical symptoms. The late phase also heightens specific sensitivity to the primary allergenic stimulus and nonspecific stimuli. Successful therapy in allergic rhinitis is the prevention or suppression of both allergic and inflammatory processes.

In affected individuals, the symptoms of repetitive sneezing, profuse rhinorrhea, chronic nasal congestion, and severe postnasal drainage can dramatically affect their lifestyles and daily activities. Treatment of these distressing symptoms includes use of topical medications: sympathomimetics, cromolyn sodium, and/or corticosteroids given intranasally or, alternatively, systemically administered antihistamines, sympathomimetics, corticosteroids, or allergen-specific immunotherapy. Each pharmacologic agent has its distinct advantages and disadvantages.

ALLERGENS

Rhinitis is a heterogeneous disease process set into motion by multiple triggering factors. Allergic rhinitis specifically can be precipitated by exposure to seasonal airborne allergens such as pollens and mold spores or by exposure to perennial allergens, such as house dust mites, cockroaches and other insect-related allergens, and animal proteins.

Indoor allergens—dust mites, fecal particles and decaying body parts—represent a significant indoor allergen burden in the home. Mites feed off dried skin debris and accumulate in mattresses, box springs, feather pillows, carpeting, stuffed animals, and wool clothing. Mite-specific growth season requirements depend on an optimal temperature (60 to 80°F) and humidity (55 to 85%). Mites represent a significant indoor burden because of our typically airtight homes with central heating and air conditioning systems that continue to circulate the allergen through the indoor air.

Cockroaches and various other insects (e.g., house flies) may also be important indoor allergens. Their salivary protein, decaying body parts, and emanations appear to be the allergenic components. These insects are most prominent in older dwellings and areas close to sea level or humid and damp locations. The allergens of smaller particle size are easily circulated through the indoor ventilation system.

Another important source for inducing indoor symptoms is animals: not only domesticated cats and dogs, but also rodents (e.g., mice, hamsters, gerbils, guinea pigs) introduced into the house as pets or reflective of poor living conditions. The allergen load actually reflects protein from three different sources—the saliva, the urine, and, primarily, the dander of the animal. A percentage of smaller (3 to 5 μm) particles stays suspended in the air for 12 to 24 hours after being disturbed, as opposed to dust mite particles, which are heavier and tend to fall to the ground after only one or two hours. Urinary protein is also the major allergen source from laboratory animals and rodents. The nocturnal patterns of these animals and their frequent location in the bedrooms of homes add to the nocturnal allergen load.

Relevance of this allergen burden is demonstrated by the child exposed nightly to allergen with a pet sleeping in his or her arms, from dust mite material in the mattress and carpeting or from urinary protein of the hamster's cage.

Outdoor pollen allergens reflect not only intact pollen grains (23 μg in diameter) but also pollen fragments (3 to 7 μm in diameter) and microaerosol suspensions of specific ragweed protein (e.g., ragweed antigen E 3 to 7 μm). A single ragweed plant produces a million grains of pollen in one day. As these pollen grains are deposited on the ground, humidity, dew, and rainfall begin to extract the relevant protein from the pollen grains, and this then becomes airborne as microaerosol particles and droplets. A similar phenomenon occurs with mold, with the dispersion into the air of not only spores, but also mycelial elements and distinct soluble protein from these mold components. Thus, a considerable burden of both perennial and seasonal allergens can impact on an allergic patient's environment.

PATHOPHYSIOLOGY

The hallmark of allergic rhinitis has been sneezing; however, rhinitis is also an inflammatory process involving mucosal edema, mucus production, and increased vascular permeability. An allergic reaction involves the specific interaction of allergen with IgE antibodies bound to receptors on mast cells and basophils. Bridging of IgE receptors leads to modification of the receptor and results in a complex sequence of biochemical events, causing cellular activation, arachidonic acid metabolism, and mediator release. Biochemical mediators so far identified include preformed mediators such as histamine, various enzymes, and chemotactic factors (important in the subsequent late phase), as well as newly generated mediators of the arachidonic acid pathway—prostaglandins (PGD_2), leukotrienes (LTC_4, LTD_4, LTE_4), and platelet-activating factor (PAF) (Figure 14-1).

The late-phase component of the allergic reaction can be observed in both the upper and lower airways. Typically, this late phase appears four to ten hours after allergen exposure and results in a recrudescence of symptoms accompanied by the generation of a second wave of inflammatory mediators. Chemotactic factors released during the immediate phase from mast cells, macrophages, and various lymphocytes are responsible for recruiting neutrophils, eosinophils, and basophils into the inflammatory site. These inflammatory cells reside at the site and begin releasing specific mediators, resulting in a smoldering late-phase reaction of mucosal and bronchial hyperreactivity. Lavage studies demonstrate that eosinophils represent the most prominent inflammatory cells present in this late phase. Furthermore, neutrophil products such as reactive oxidants and enzymes may also contribute to this inflammatory damage in the airways. This inflammation induces a heightened response to repeated exposure to the specific allergen (termed "priming") as well as the development of a heightened sensitivity to nonspecific irritants (e.g., pollutants, smoke, perfumes, cold air).

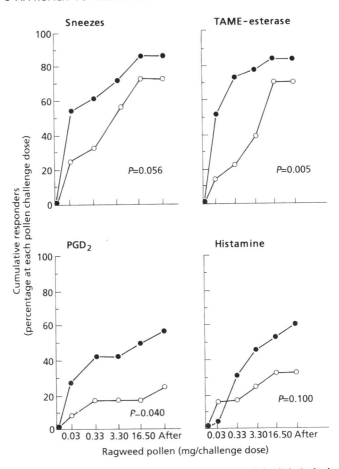

Figure 14-1. Comparison of nontreated (*n* = 26) (solid circles) and treated (*n* = 12) (open circles) groups of patients based on cumulative percentage of patients sneezing or demonstrating mediator release at each respective pollen challenge dose. Statistical comparison made on threshold dose of pollen required to provoke significant response. Reproduced with permission from Creticos PS, Adkinson Jr NF, Kagey-Sobotka A, et al. Nasal challenge with ragweed pollen in hay fever patients. J Clin Invest 1985;76:2247–2253.

DIAGNOSTIC APPROACH

Evaluation of the rhinitis patient should include a thorough history, with particular attention to those environmental factors in the house, work, or outdoor setting that could influence the allergic process. Identification of specific triggering factors coupled with appropriate environmental manipulation can have a dramatic impact. The diagnostic approach should incorporate a carefully selected skin test evaluation both to determine whether an allergic component of the disease process exists and, if so, to provide accurate data on the degree of clinical sensitivity. In selected individuals, a radioallergosorbent test (RAST) can also provide useful data.

The management of allergic rhinitis logically hinges on instituting appropriate anti-inflammatory therapy with topical nasal steroids or cromolyn to suppress the inflammatory component with the addition of antihistamines and/or decongestants to treat acute or breakthrough symptoms.

PATIENT EDUCATION

Educating patients is the most crucial component of any therapeutic plan. Patient education includes reviewing the plan of action with the patient, discussing the proper use of medications and their side effects, and making sure the patient knows when to call or see the physician or staff. Understanding the reasoning behind the use of the medications on a daily basis and learning how to adjust medications to control minor "breakthroughs" are necessary both to ensure compliance and to prevent worsening of disease.

PHARMACOTHERAPY: ANTIHISTAMINES

Antihistamines play an important role in the treatment of allergic rhinitis. They relieve acute, intermittent symptoms as well as providing long-term management of persistent symptoms. Antihistamines are competitive antagonists to histamine for H_1 receptor sites on target cells. Classic antihistamines possess ethylamine moieties similar in structure to histamine itself, whereas the newer antihistamines are piperazine- or piperidine-like compounds with tricyclic ringed structures that may account for the properties unique to these therapeutic agents.

Classic antihistamines are highly lipophilic and easily penetrate the central nervous system (CNS), whereas the newer agents are relatively lipophobic and cross the blood-brain barrier only poorly; hence, they are classified as nonsedating. Furthermore, second and third generation antihistamines appear to be able to inhibit the release of inflammatory mediators from the mast cell, a property not shared by classic antihistamines. This ability suggests that anti-histamines, in addition to treating acute symptoms, may also con-tribute to dampening the entire allergic inflammatory cascade (by mast cell stabilization). Clinical implications of this inhibition are intriguing since antihistamines typically have no appreciable effect on nasal congestion. This expands the potential therapeutic appli-cation of third-generation antihistamines to include not only simple histamine antagonism but also an ability to turn off the inflamma-tory response in both the upper and lower airways through their anti-inflammatory properties.

Side effects of antihistamines

Because the first-generation compounds freely penetrate the CNS, these agents produce significant drowsiness and fatigue in 10 to 25% of patients. More importantly, first-generation antihistamines may interfere with the ability to perform tasks that require motor skills, such as driving a car or operating machinery. Furthermore, in some patients, especially the elderly, these antihistamines may also cause troublesome anticholinergic side effects, such as difficulty with urination, impotence, or dryness of the mouth. In addition, a smaller number of patients may complain of gastrointestinal discomfort such as queasiness or nausea. In high enough doses, adverse cardiovascular effects can also be induced by the first-generation and second-generation antihistamines, ranging from palpitations through superventricular tachycardias to ventricular disturbances (Torsade des pointes).

Advantages of the new second-generation antihistamines

In contrast, the second-generation antihistamines have several ad-vantages (Table 14-1). The most obvious reason for choosing them

---

Table 14-1. Second-Generation Antihistamines

Lipophobic
Highly protein bound
Effective H_1-receptor antagonism
Lack anticholinergic activity
Minimal sedation
Little performance impairment
Cardiovascular event—drug interaction

---

is the lack of sedation. More importantly, the second-generation antihistamines do not interfere with the ability to perform motor tasks. Neither terfenadine nor loratadine interferes with the subject's ability to perform a simulated driving performance test, whereas the classic sedating first-generation antihistamine triprolidine impaired driving skills in study subjects for up to four hours, and this impairment was comparable to that seen in drivers with a blood-alcohol concentration of 0.05% (Figure 14-2).

Adverse effects of the second-generation antihistamines

Recently, information has become available regarding the risk of the second-generation antihistamines in causing cardiac arrhythmias which, although rare, have led to fatal and near-fatal outcomes. These events were first noted in patients taking an accidental overdose or in patients attempting suicide. However, it is also apparent that there are certain clinical settings that predispose patients to the development of adverse cardiovascular events (underlying hepatic disease, specific drug interactions, certain cardiovascular settings).

Underlying liver disease can impair the metabolism of antihistamines that depend upon the cytochrome p450 enzyme systems for their breakdown. This impairment can lead to toxic blood levels, which could result in adverse cardiovascular events.

The potential for drug interaction is present with any medication and is further complicated for a patient taking multiple drugs. Concomitant administration of terfenadine and astemizole is contraindicated in patients taking certain macrolide antibiotics (e.g., erythromycin) or antifungal agents (e.g., oral ketoconazole or itraconazole). The potential for the interaction of these second-generation antihistamines with other macrolide antibiotics or other antifungals should not be overlooked.

The third possibility involves underlying cardiovascular disease, which could predispose to serious arrhythmias. This becomes particularly relevant in those situations where the Q-T interval can be prolonged since the second-generation antihistamines have been demonstrated to prolong the Q-T interval and thereby induce ventricular tachyarrythmias. In this context, these antihistamines should be avoided in patients with known prolongation of the Q-T interval, in patients with underlying hypomagnesemia or hypokalemia or other conditions that predispose the Q-T interval prolongation, in patients with underlying ventricular tachyarrhythmia, and in patients currently receiving class 1A

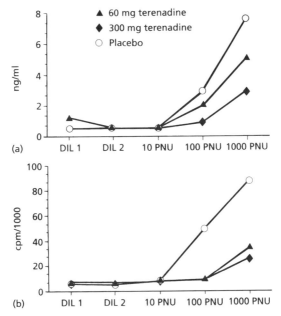

Figure 14-2. In a double-blind study 12 patients with allergic rhinitis were pretreated for one week with terfenadine 60 mg two times daily or terfenadine 300 mg two times daily and then challenged intranasally, out of season, with an antigen to which they had been naturally sensitized. Median levels of (a) histamine and (b) TAME-esterase activity are shown in recovered nasal voyages after antigen challenge. The nasal challenge protocol is our own on the abscissa. DIL, Diluent for antigen extract; PNU, protein nitrogen units; open circles represent the response after placebo pretreatment; closed triangles and diamonds represent the responses after 1 week's pretreatment with terfenadine 60 mg two times daily or terfenadine 300 mg two times daily, repectively. Terfenadine, but not placebo, inhibited the release of histamine and TAME-esterase activity. Reproduced with permission from Naclerio RM, Kagey-Sobotka A, Lichtenstein LM, et al. The effect of cetirizine on early allergy response. Laryngoscope 1989;99:596–599.

antiarrhythmic drugs such as quinidine, procainamide, and disopyramide that, in and of themselves, lead to Q-T prolongation.

This risk of potentially fatal ventricular arrhythmias should be put in perspective. Given the large number of patients who have taken second-generation antihistamines around the world (>200,000,000 patient-months of use) the relevant risk of such events is rare. With careful attention to a patient's clinical history, the practitioner can prescribe the second-generation antihistamines, terfenadine and astemizole, for the appropriate patient. The development of newer second-generation antihistamines, loratadine, fexofenadine, and cetirizine, has largely overcome this problem. The recommended dose of any antihistamine should not be exceeded. It is important to stress the proper way to take the medication to the patient.

Clinical efficacy

Numerous double-blind, placebo-controlled studies have demonstrated the effectiveness of antihistamines in the treatment of allergic rhinoconjunctivitis. Second-generation antihistamines are as effective as a "classic" antihistamine, chlorpheniramine (4mg three times a day), in relieving sneezing and rhinorrhea, yet their control of nasal congestion was poor. As would be expected, the incidence of drowsiness with the first-generation antihistamine was significantly greater than that experienced in the terfenadine-treated group (in one study, 19% versus 7.6%).

Several studies have compared the second-generation antihistamines terfenadine, cetirizine, and loratadine, which have shown comparable relief in both seasonal and perennial rhinitis. Sneezing, rhinorrhea, itchy nose and throat, and eye symptoms were more effectively controlled with astemizole, 10mg a day, than with terfenadine, 60mg twice a day. Neither drug was any more effective than placebo in controlling nasal congestion. A number of studies have compared cetirizine with terfenadine or astemizole; the antihistamines appear to be equally effective for control of sneezing; itchy nose, throat, and palate; eye symptoms; and nasal congestion; however, cetirizine appeared to be more effective at improving rhinorrhea.

Conclusion

Antihistamines are an effective therapeutic choice for relief of intermittent or mild symptoms of allergic rhinoconjunctivitis. In more persistent or moderately severe disease, their role as an adjunctive medication in conjunction with inhaled corticosteroids or cromolyn is often essential for the most effective management of seasonal or perennial allergic rhinitis. The new second-generation antihistamines, such as astemizole, terfenadine, and loratadine, are safe and effective nonsedating medications with properties that should enhance patient compliance.

PHARMACOTHERAPY: CROMOLYN

Cromolyn is a derivative of khellin, a naturally occurring antispasmodic extracted from the Mediterranean plant Ammi visnaga, or "Bishop's Weed." The mechanisms of cromolyn's action are not completely understood: it appears that one action may be to stabilize mast cell membranes and inhibit the subsequent release of mediators associated with the allergic reaction. The importance of this inhibitory function is demonstrated by cromolyn preventing the immediate phase of an allergic reaction. In addition to blocking the early-phase response, cromolyn is also capable of blocking the late phase of the allergic reaction. Cromolyn has the ability to interfere with various chemotactic factors responsible for recruiting cells (eosinophils, neutrophils, and basophils) into the inflammatory site, and hence abrogate the late-phase reaction.

Clinical efficacy

Clinical studies have demonstrated the efficacy of cromolyn applied topically to the nasal mucosa for the treatment of both seasonal and perennial rhinitis (Figure 14-3). However, to be optimally effective, cromolyn requires judicious use on a daily basis by the patient. An aggressive therapeutic regimen is started with two sprays three or four times a day, and may take one to two weeks to achieve optimal results. After symptom control is achieved, taper the drug to one or two sprays in each nostril one to three times a day as long-term therapy.

The most important key to successful therapy with cromolyn is to employ the medication prophylactically. To perform this, cromolyn should be started seven to ten days prior to the anticipated allergen season or allergen exposure as one or two sprays in each nostril four times a day for one to two weeks. This approach requires patient compliance, but with proper education, the therapeutic benefit of cromolyn should take effect. Cromolyn can be tapered to a more convenient regimen of one to three times a day to sustain relief. Experience with cromolyn bears out that 60 to 70% of patients who adhere to the prescribed dosage regimens will obtain very good to excellent results (Figure 14-4).

Ophthalmic preparations of cromolyn have also been shown to be effective in the treatment of seasonal allergic conjunctivitis, giant papillary conjunctivitis, atopic keratoconjunctivitis, and vernal keratoconjunctivitis. In these situations, the standard ophthalmic dosage is one or two drops in each eye every four hours until

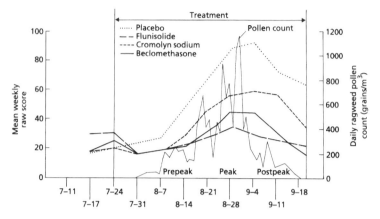

Figure 14-3. Mean weekly raw scores for symptoms of hay fever among 120 patients in four study groups, based on treatment: placebo, cromolyn sodium (Nasalcrom), flunisolide (Nasalide), and beclomethasone nasal solution (Beconase AQ). Study was conducted during ragweed season in 1984. Daily ragweed pollen count is shown in enclosed area. See text for details of derivation of hay-fever score. All active treatments were more effective than placebo, and the two glucocorticoids were more effective than cromolyn in preventing symptoms of hay fever. Reproduced with permission from Welsh PW, Strickler WE, Chu CP, et al. Efficacy of beclomethasone nasal solution, flunisolide, and cromolyn in relieving symptoms of ragweed allergy. Mayo Clin Proc 1987;62:125–134.

symptoms are controlled, then one or two drops in each eye two to four times a day. Symptom control is usually observed within two to three days, probably reflecting the fact that the conjunctival mucosa is more easily saturated by the ophthalmic preparation as compared to the nasal mucosal surfaces. Other ophthalmic preparations useful for allergic conjunctivitis are lodoxamide 0.1%, ketorolac 0.5%, levocabastine 0.05%, and naphazoline 0.025%, combined with pheniramine 0.3%. Lodoxamide is very similar to cromolyn in its effect on mast cell degranulation. Ketorolac is a nonsteroidal anti-inflammatory agent. Levocabastine and pheniramine are antihistamines, while naphazoline is a vasoconstrictor.

Comparative studies have generally shown cromolyn sodium to be comparable, if not superior, to antihistamines in the relief of allergic rhinitis. This conclusion should be balanced by the observation that cromolyn more effectively controls nasal congestion

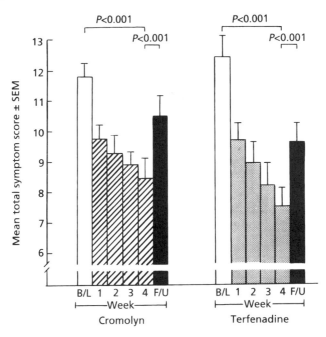

Figure 14-4. In a randomized double-blind study, patients with allergic rhinitis received either cromolyn 4% solution, one puff in each nostril four times daily, or terfenadine 60 mg two times daily, along with the appropriate placebo spray or tablet for 4 weeks, following a 1-week baseline qualification period. Mean ±SEM total symptom scores at baseline, at the end of each week of therapy, and at follow-up visit after 1 week without therapy are shown. The P values are for differences between means within treatments. Cromolyn and terfenadine were comparably effective and well-accepted treatments for allergic rhinitis. Reproduced with permission from Orgel HA, Meltzer EO, Kemp JP, Ostrom NK, Welch MJ. Comparison of intranasal cromolyn sodium, 4%, and oral terfenadine for allergic rhinitis: symptoms, nasal cytology, nasal ciliary clearance, and rhinomanometry. Ann Allergy 1991;66:237–244.

while antihistamines provide generally more effective relief of ocular symptoms. Both groups demonstrated significant and comparable improvement in the severity of allergic rhinitis over the course of the four-week treatment period, as compared to their baseline symptomatology. No major side effects were noted in either group. In this regard, total nasal symptoms were more effectively controlled by beclomethasone than by terfenadine, especially during the peak grass pollen period; however, beclomethasone did not provide as effective relief of eye symptoms as did the antihistamine.

In conclusion, cromolyn is an effective anti-inflammatory therapeutic agent for the treatment of seasonal and perennial rhinoconjunctivitis. However, to be optimally effective, it must be used on a daily basis.

Adverse effects

Cromolyn appears to exert its actions topically at or within the mucosal surfaces. Studies demonstrate that less than 7% of the total administered dose of nasal cromolyn is absorbed across the human nasal mucosa. This absorbed drug is rapidly excreted and changed in the bile and the urine. The clinical studies noted above showed that cromolyn was well tolerated by patients with only nasal irritation or burning reported. There was no evidence of septal perforation or ulceration in patients treated with cromolyn.

TOPICAL GLUCOCORTICOSTEROIDS

Topical inhaled steroid preparations exert their effects through a number of different mechanisms to suppress IgE-mediated allergic inflammation. On a cellular level, these compounds penetrate the cell and bind to specific receptors within the cell to alter messenger RNA in subsequent protein expression. Their effects include inhibition of mediator synthesis of the arachidonic-acid pathway, inhibition of leukocyte migration, and downregulation of the effects of various mediators on their target cells at the tissue level.

Utilizing the nasal challenge model, it has been demonstrated that topical application of glucocorticosteroids can not only suppress the late phase of the allergic reaction, but also significantly attenuate the early-phase immediate allergic response. The effects of topical application of flunisolide $200\,\mu g/day$ applied for seven days prior to allergy challenge in 13 allergic patients showed a reduction in symptoms of sneezing and inflammatory mediators characteristic of the allergic response. In contrast, oral prednisone only mitigates the late phase of reactivity and has no effect on immediate allergic response. The importance of corticosteroids is borne out in our approach to management of the patient with allergic disease. Using a topical anti-inflammatory preparation on a daily basis suppresses the inflammatory component.

The topical steroid preparations currently available for nasal therapy include beclomethasone, budesonide, dexamethamosone, flunisolide, fluticasone, and triamcinolone (Table 14-2). Studies suggest that doses between 200 and 400 μg/day provide very good to excellent results in 70 to 85% of patients treated. Efficacy has been demonstrated in seasonal allergic rhinitis, perennial allergic rhinitis, nonallergic rhinitis with eosinophilia (NARES), chronic rhinitis (presumably with a predominant nonallergic basis), and chronic rhinitis associated with nasal polyposis (Figures 14-5 and 14-6).

Clinical efficacy with topical nasal steroid preparations has been demonstrated within three to four days of instituting therapy and was maintained over the duration of treatment.

Comparative studies

Comparative studies of antihistamines and inhaled steroids consistently favor the inhaled steroid when the adequate daily dose regimen is complied with. However, one obvious difference is appreciated in that eye symptoms conversely are not as well controlled with a topical nasal steroid preparation as compared to a systemic oral antihistamine.

Many studies have compared the effects of nasal steroids to aqueous cromolyn in the management of ragweed-induced fall pollenosis (Figure 14-7). The topical steroid preparations provided comparable efficacy, which was superior to that of cromolyn. An interesting corollary to this study was that aggressive treatment of upper airway symptoms not only modified the symptoms of allergic rhinitis, but also mitigated lower airway symptoms as manifested by the need for asthma bronchodilator medications in the groups of patients in active therapy with topical nasal steroid preparations.

Table 14-2.   Nasal Corticosteroid Preparations

Dexamethasone phosphate
Beclomethasone dipropionate
Flunisolide
Triamcinolone acetonide
Fluticasone propionate
Budesonide

235

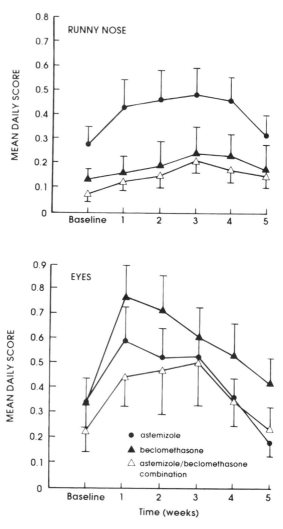

Figure 14-5. In a randomized double-blind parallel-group trial, 90 patients with allergic rhinitis received either beclomethasone dipropionate aqueous nasal spray 400 µg daily or astemizole 10 mg daily, or both medications daily. Treatment was started 1 week before the ragweed pollen season and continued daily until 1 week after the season, for a total of 6 weeks. Patients taking beclomethasone alone had significantly less sneezing, nasal obstruction, and rhinorrhea, and required less "rescue" medication than patients taking astemizole alone. Beclomethasone plus astemizole provided no better control of nasal symptoms than beclomethasone alone. Eye symptoms and "rescue" eye drop use

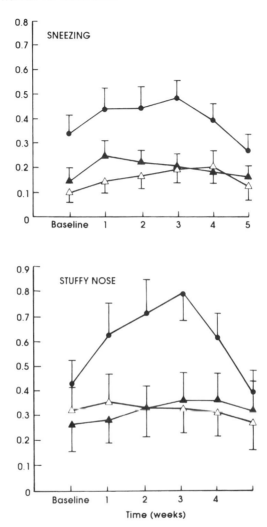

Figure 14-5. *Continued* tended to be less in patients taking astemizole alone than in patients taking beclomethasone alone, but the best control of eye symptoms was recorded in patients taking both medications. Reproduced with permission from Juniper EF, Kline PA, Hargreave FE, Dolorich J. Comparison of beclomethasone dipropionate aqueous nasal spray, astemizole, and the combination in the prophylactic treatment of ragweed pollen–induced rhinoconjunctivitis. J Allergy Clin Immunol 1989;83: 627–633.

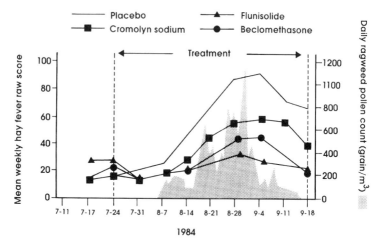

Figure 14-6. In a randomized blinded parallel-group study, 120 patients with allergic rhinitis received either beclomethasone aqueous solution, 0.5% two times daily (336 µg/day), flunisolide nasal solution 0.025% two times daily (200 µg/day), cromolyn nasal solution 4% four times daily (41.6 mg/day), or placebo during the ragweed pollen season. Beclomethasone, flunisolide, and cromolyn provided better control of symptoms than placebo ($P < 0.001$). The two inhaled glucocorticoids were significantly more effective than cromolyn ($P < 0.001$). In this study, all active intranasal treatments also significantly reduced the symptoms of seasonal asthma (data not shown). Reproduced with permission from Welsh PW, Strickler WE, Chu CP, et al. Efficacy of beclomethasone nasal solution, flunisolide, and cromolyn in relieving symptoms of ragweed allergy. Mayo Clin Proc 1987;62:125–134.

Side effects

In the doses typically required to control nasal symptoms (200 to 400 µg/day), topical steroid preparations are not associated with systemic corticosteroid side effects. The major complaints by patients are nasal burning, nasal stinging, and nasal irritation. In a previously traumatized nose (e.g., cauterization/prior surgery with disruption of the vascular bed), nasal perforation may occur. Nasal ulceration and/or perforation can occur when the patient with rhinitis uses the nasal corticosteroid improperly. For instance, this could occur with improper use of the applicator, where mechanical trauma from the device impinges on the septal wall, causing an erosion leading to an ulceration and, rarely, to a perforation.

Multiple studies have determined A.M. cortisol levels, 17-hydroxycorticosteroid level in the urine, or incorporated stimula-

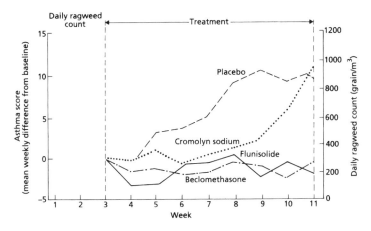

Figure 14-7. A tenfold decrease in asthma symptom scores was reported during the peak ragweed season by patients with rhinitis who received intranasal flunisolide or beclomethasone, compared with placebo. During this period, intranasal cromolyn sodium reduced asthma symptom scores by threefold over placebo. These results suggest that managing rhinitis improves asthma symptoms in patients with concurrent disease. Reproduced with permission from Welsh PW, Strickler WE, Chu CP, et al. Efficacy of beclomethasone nasal solution, flunisolide, and cromolyn in relieving symptoms of ragweed allergy. Mayo Clin Proc 1987;62:125–134.

tion tests for adrenal suppression. The consensus from these studies suggests that in children adrenal suppression would not be expected until a dose of greater than 800 µg of beclomethasone (or its equivalent) is administered; and in adults this would not be expected until a dose of greater than 1200 to 1500 µg is applied topically on a daily basis.

Summary

Our approach to the patient with persistent symptoms of allergic rhinitis should be to employ a topical anti-inflammatory therapeutic agent (e.g., a topical group of corticoids of cromolyn) in an attempt to suppress the inflammatory response. To be most effective, these medications should be begun prophylactically or, if started in presently symptomatic patients, must be used on a regular daily basis to achieve success. Concomitantly, antihistamines should be employed for breakthrough symptoms of itchy, watery eyes, runny nose, and sneezing, and/or decongestants should be administered for nasal congestion and stuffiness. Certainly, in many patients, optimal therapy requires employing a combination of these therapeutic agents to achieve optimal success.

ANTICHOLINERGIC AGENTS

Atropine sulfate was originally used 100 years ago for nasal coryza and rhinorrhea caused by allergic rhinitis. The topical potency of atropine has subsequently been studied as a treatment of obstructive airway diseases. Unfortunately, the systemic and drying side effects of atropine have limited its use in asthma even though it has a definite bronchodilator action.

Alternatively, atropine is used as an active ingredient in cough–cold preparations in order to reduce excessive secretions from the nose and eyes. Oral doses of 0.2 to 0.3 mg of atropine sulfate are probably safe, but there is insufficient data to establish atropine's effectiveness.

In prior studies, atropine as a 1 mg/ml solution is effective in studies reducing rhinorrhea caused by allergic rhinitis (seven patients) or viral-induced rhinitis (24 patients). All patients except one reported substantial reduction in nasal secretions. Three out of 31 patients had obvious vasoconstriction of nasal blood vessels, whereas none of the subjects reported dry mouth or visual disturbances. Atropine's duration of action was noted to be three to four hours and longer in five patients observed for longer periods of time. Two studies using 0.025% nasal solution (400 μg/day for four weeks) show no serious adverse effects but little difference from placebo in controlling mild to severe symptoms of rhinorrhea.

Other studies of anticholinergic agents for rhinitis have focused upon the quaternary salt of ipratropium. These and other studies have demonstrated efficacy in reducing nasal secretions in both allergic and nonallergic rhinitis, indicating that the cholinergic receptor is important in the control of nasal secretions. The side-effect profile also shows just local adverse drying but no serious systemic side effects compatible with an anticholinergic agent. Surprisingly these studies have not noted any effect on sneezing, nasal congestion, or itching. This lack of effect suggests that cholinergic receptors have only a minimal role in causing these chronic rhinitis symptoms.

SELECTED REFERENCES

Andersson M, Andersson P, Pipkorn U. Topical glucocorticosteroids and allergen-induced increase in nasal reactivity: relationship between treatment time and inhibitory effect. J Allergy Clin Immunol 1988;82:1019–1026.

Anggard A, Lundberg JM, Lundblad L. Nasal autonomic innervation with special reference to peptidergic nerves. Eur J Respir Dis 1983;64(suppl 128):143–148.

Bascom R, Wachs M, Naclerio RM, et al. Basophil influx occurs after nasal antigen challenge: effects of topical corticosteroid pretreatment. J Allergy Clin Immunol 1988;81:580–589.

Bisgaard H. Leukotrienes and prostaglandins in asthma. Allergy 1984;39:413–420.

Connell JT. Quantitative intranasal pollen challenge—Effect of a daily pollen challenge, environmental pollen exposure, and placebo challenge on the nasal membrane. J Allergy 1968;41:123–139.

Franklin W. Perennial rhinitis. In: McKay I, ed. Rhinitis. Mechanisms and management. Suffolk: William Clowes, 1989:117–140.

Georgitis JW, Banov C, Boggs PB, et al. Ipratropium bromide nasal spray in non-allergic rhinitis: efficacy, nasal cytological response and patient evaluation on quality of life. Clin Exp Allergy 1994;24:1049–1055.

Klementsson J, Andersson M, Pipkorn U. Allergen-induced increase in nonspecific nasal reactivity is blocked by antihistamines without a clear-cut relationship to eosinophil influx. J Allergy Clin Immunol 1990;86:466–472.

Meltzer EO, Orgel HA, Bronsky EA, et al. Ipratropium bromide aqueous nasal spray for patients with perennial allergic rhinitis: a study of its effect on their symptoms, quality of life, and nasal cytology. J Allergy Clin Immunol 1992;90:242–249.

Middleton E. Chronic rhinitis in adults. J Allergy Clin Immunol 1988;81:971–975.

Mygind N. Essential allergy. Oxford: Blackwell Scientific Publications, 1986:279–350.

Naclerio RM, Meier HL, Kagey-Sobotka A, et al. Mediator release after nasal airway challenge with allergen. Am Rev Respir Dis 1983;128:597–602.

Norman PS. Allergic rhinitis. In: Frank MM, Austen KF, Claman HN, Unnanue ER, eds. Samter's Immunologic Diseases, 5th ed. Boston: Little, Brown, 1995:1273–1282.

Orgel HA, Meltzer EO, Kemp JP, et al. Comparison of intranasal cromolyn sodium, 4%, and oral terfenadine for allergic rhinitis: symptoms, nasal cytology, nasal ciliary clearance, and rhinomanometry. Ann Allergy 1991;66:237–244.

Pipkorn U, Proud D, Lichtenstein LM, et al. Inhibition of mediator release in allergic rhinitis by pretreatment with topical glucocorticosteroids. N Engl J Med 1987;316:1506–1510.

Pipkorn U, Pukander J, Suonpaa J, et al. Long-term safety of budesonide nasal aerosol: 15-year follow-up study. Clin Allergy 1988;18:253–259.

Simons FER, Simons KJ. Antihistamines: H_1 and H_2-receptor antagonists. In: Middleton EM Jr, Reed CE, Ellis EF, et al., eds. Allergy: principles and practice. St Louis: C.V. Mosby, 1992:856–892.

Togias A, Naclerio RM, Proud D, et al. Studies on the allergic and nonallergic nasal inflammation. J Allergy Clin Immunol 1988;81:782–790.

Van Cauwenberge P. Epidemiology of common cold. Rhinology 1985;23:273–282.

Van Cauwenberge P, Tyberghein J. Differential diagnosis of rhinopathy. Acta Otorhinolaryngol Belg 1979;33:537–614.

Welsh PW, Stricker WE, Chu C-P, et al. Efficacy of beclomethasone nasal solution, flunisolide, and cromolyn in relieving symptoms of ragweed allergy. Mayo Clinic Proc 1987;62:125–134.

Immunotherapy for Upper Airway Disorders

15

INTRODUCTION

Immunotherapy can be highly successful for aeroallergen-induced allergic airway disorders such as allergic rhinitis and allergic asthma. Immunotherapy is best described as slow immunization to a specific aeroallergen or allergens, yet it has intrinsic risks associated with the treatments. Obviously the patient must manifest symptoms after allergen exposure and have demonstrable allergen-specific IgE by either skin testing or serological testing before utilizing immunotherapy for the disorder.

Allergic airway diseases, rhinitis and asthma, are fairly common and chronic disorders. Allergic rhinitis by conservative estimates affects at least 20% of the general population. An additional 7 to 10% of people can develop allergic rhinitis over the years. Allergic rhinitis classically affects people in their peak productive years of 10 to 35 years but can affect infants and the elderly. There is a high morbidity and cost associated with allergic rhinitis: $500 million per year in health care costs, 2 million lost school days, 3.5 million lost work days, and 2.8 million days in restricted activity. Allergic rhinitis is also associated with other disorders such as chronic or recurrent sinusitis, acute and chronic otitis media, asthma, and atopic dermatitis. In fact, 20% of rhinitis patients also have asthma.

Asthma is thought to affect 5% of the population or more than 10 million Americans. It is a far more serious disorder, since mortality rates are rising nationally and internationally in select populations. Costs for treatment for asthma were $3.6 billion in 1990 for hospital and physician expenses and $1.1 billion in medications. The indirect expenses for asthma were $2.6 billion, which includes lost school days and days absent from work. Allergy is one of many triggers for asthma and may be the major cause for underlying bronchial hyperreactivity present in asthma. Of note, 60% of asthmatics also suffer with concurrent rhinitis symptoms.

Most treatments for allergic airway disorders are palliative and consist of antihistamines, sympathomimetics (decongestants), mast cell stabilizers (cromolyn sodium), and corticosteroids for chronic rhinitis; for asthma, bronchodilators (β_2-agonists), phosphodiesterase inhibitors (theophylline), anticholinergics (ipratropium bromide), mast cell stabilizers (cromolyn and nedocromil), and corticosteroids. Immunotherapy addresses the underlying allergic reaction and attempts to modify the response to aeroallergens that induce the reaction.

Aeroallergens include pollens, molds, and animal particles and products, such as hair, saliva, dander, urine, feces, and body parts (mammals, mites, birds, insects). An aeroallergen must be sensitizing and be present in the ambient air in ample quantities to cause symptoms in an allergic individual. Ragweed pollen is probably the most cited example of an aeroallergen in that people allergic to ragweed have significant exposure during the months of August and September.

MECHANISMS OF IMMUNOTHERAPY

Several general principles must be taken into consideration before instituting immunotherapy. Obviously, the patient needs to be highly sensitive. IgE-mediated sensitivity should be documented to a specific aeroallergen by either cutaneous testing or in vitro testing. There also needs to be an extract of the aeroallergen. Immunotherapy needs to be given in relatively high doses for a long time. The dose must be close to the dose that produces local and systemic reactions. A favorable response is a reduction in symptoms.

Effective immunotherapy alters skin test response, basophil histamine release, release of mediators into nasal secretions during challenge, and bronchial reactivity (Figure 15-1). The favorable clinical effect is often seen before alteration of these immunologic findings. The clinical response is often associated with an increase in allergen-specific IgG identified as "blocking antibody." There are, however, exceptions, where some patients have a favorable response but no IgG antibody production. With immunotherapy,

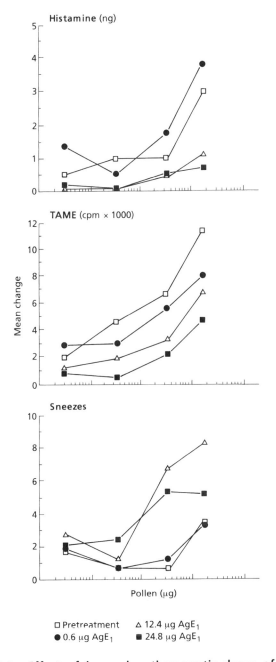

Figure 15-1. Effect of increasing therapeutic doses of ragweed immunotherapy (0.6, 12.4, 24.8 µg AgE) on nasal challenge response in 11 patients. Dose–response curves demonstrate the mean of the increases from prechallenge levels for histamine, TAME, and sneezes. Vertical axis plots the mean change in mediator; horizontal axis, dose of pollen challenge. Reprinted from Busse WW, Holgate ST. Asthma and Rhinitis. Boston: Blackwell Science, 1995.

there is an initial rise in serum allergen-specific IgE, then blunting of the seasonal rise in IgE and ultimately a fall in IgE titers. Immunotherapy may also reduce mast cell sensitivity to aeroallergens independent of its effects on B cell production of IgE and IgG.

The rationale for immunotherapy is that in nature, avoidance of pollens, molds, and house dust mites is extremely difficult and unrealistic at times. Alternatively, some aeroallergens such as animal danders from dogs or cats and urine from laboratory animals can be avoided. The goal of immunotherapy is to increase the patient's tolerance to natural exposure of the aeroallergen resulting in symptom control and decrease in medication use.

Efficacy of immunotherapy for allergic rhinitis has been well documented, starting with the initial studies by Frankland and Augustin, Lowell and Franklin, and Norman and coworkers. In placebo-controlled trials, ragweed immunotherapy demonstrated efficacy based upon symptom–medication scores. This effect was dose-related; maintenance doses of $1\,\mu g$ or more of antigen E (Amb a I) were effective, and lower doses ranging from 0.00024 to $0.006\,\mu g$ were ineffective. Other immunologic findings include a rise in serum IgG, an initial rise in serum IgE and then a decline to pretreatment levels, no seasonal rise in IgE, an increase in ragweed-specific IgA and IgG in nasal secretions, a decrease in lymphocyte responsiveness to ragweed, an increase in threshold allergen dose on nasal challenge for release of inflammatory mediators (histamine, PGD_2, leukotrienes, and kinins), and suppression of late-phase skin reactions to intradermal ragweed extract (Figures 15-2 and 15-3). Similar double-blind studies have shown clinical efficacy for grass, mountain cedar, and house dust mite immunotherapy.

Efficacy for allergic asthma is not as extensive as for rhinitis, in that aeroallergen–induced asthma often has other complicating factors such as irritants, exercise, or emotional upset causing wheezing. One study was unable to identify adequate numbers of patients to investigate ragweed immunotherapy in asthma. In grass–sensitive asthmatics given immunotherapy, two studies (Frankland and Augustin, Ortolani and associates) noted a reduction in symptoms with treatment.

Cat-induced asthma has been the best model for allergic asthma. In elegant studies, cat immunotherapy was shown to be as safe as ragweed immunotherapy. Double-blind trials using cat immunotherapy demonstrated a decrease in bronchial reactivity to cat dander, a reduction in skin prick test response, an increase in IgG

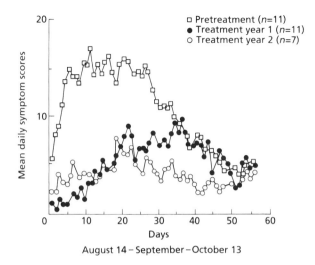

Figure 15-2. Nasal challenge model: effect of immunotherapy. Reproduced with permission from Creticos PS, Marsh DG, Proud D, et al. Responses to ragweed pollen nasal challenge before and after immunotherapy. J Allergy Clin Immunol 1989;84:197–205.

to the major cat allergen, Fel D I, and the expected response of an initial rise in IgE then fall to pretreatment levels. One study by Ohman and associates used deliberate exposure to cats in a confined area to demonstrate that patients on active immunotherapy had a significant delay before onset of eye and pulmonary symptoms. Similar studies have shown efficacy for dog immunotherapy in asthma.

Immunotherapy to house dust–induced asthma has had conflicting results, with two positive studies and one negative study. This is not surprising since house dust contains a variety of allergens ranging from mites, cockroaches, and the dander of cats, dogs, and other animals to pollens and molds. Immunotherapy to house dust mite shows a significant decrease in asthma symptoms, decrease in medications, and decrease in response to both immediate and late-phase responses during bronchoprovocation.

There are, however, immunotherapy procedures that are not effective. Low-dose regimens (Rinkel technique) have been proven ineffective in several double-blind, placebo-controlled studies. Immunotherapy based on provocation–neutralization and sublingual immunotherapy have not undergone the rigors of placebo-

247

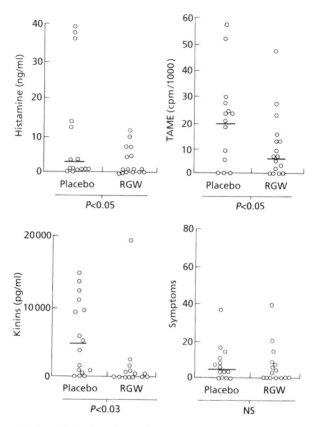

Figure 15-3. Clinical and mediator response to immunotherapy: late phase. Reproduced with permission from Fliopoulos O, Proud D, Adkinson Jr NF, et al. Effects of immunotherapy on the early, late, and rechallenge nasal reaction to provocation with allergen: changes in inflammatory mediators and cells. J Allergy Clin Immunoel 1991;87:855–860.

controlled, double-blind investigations as have other immunotherapy regimens, so the efficacy of these types is purely anecdotal.

IMMUNOTHERAPY REGIMENS

There are certain basic requirements for immunotherapy. Patients need to have symptoms of allergic rhinitis or asthma, demonstrate

IgE by skin testing or in vitro testing, and be unable to control symptoms through avoidance and/or medication. Immunotherapy should be used with other general treatment regimens (i.e., continuing asthma medications and controlling the environment).

A practical consideration is limiting the allergens to six to ten for each treatment vial. Therefore, the testing should identify the selective aeroallergens to be used for the individual. Treatment with irrelevant allergens is not advised, is wasteful, and may induce sensitivity to that allergen.

Allergenic extracts require careful storage in order to maintain their potency. Extracts lose 50% of their initial potency when kept at room temperature or by going through repeated freezing and thawing. Extracts containing 50% glycerin are stable for three years at 4°C, as are freeze-dried extracts kept at the same temperature. Concentrated aqueous extracts without glycerin stored at 4°C lose their potency slowly, so that they are at 50% potency after six months. Diluted aqueous extracts lose potency more rapidly. Use of standardized extracts is highly desirable, and the FDA now utilizes the allergy unit (AU) to characterize these extracts. For other extracts, the old method for extracts utilizes protein nitrogen units (PNU) or weight per volume (w/v).

Administration of allergenic extracts involves injection into the subcutaneous tissue of the posterior aspect of the upper arm. Commonly, a disposable tuberculin syringe with either a 26- or 27-gauge 1/2″ to 5/8″ needle is used for the injections.

The recommended starting dose for sensitive patients is 0.5 AU, 0.4 PNU, or 0.1 ml of a 1:200,000 w/v dilution. Doses may be safely increased by two-fold dilutions at weekly or twice-weekly intervals. If local or systemic reactions occur, the dose should be reduced to the previously tolerated dose. Rush or clustered schedules have been developed to expedite the immunization process but have not undergone extensive trials for aeroallergen use.

The maintenance dose is that concentration resulting in clinical reduction of symptoms and administered safely without systemic reactions. This is usually an individual response, but most patients can achieve a dose of 1000 AU—except for cat, in which case it is 25,000 AU. The interval of maintenance doses is three to four weeks. The duration of therapy is dictated by the patient but is commonly two to three years, during which there is gradual clinical symptom control. Discontinuation of immunotherapy may be considered after this interval, weighing the risk of reappearance of symptoms. In situations without clinical improvement, one must consider either modification of the immunotherapy or cessation of the regimen.

Most patients on immunotherapy experience local reactions such as localized swelling and erythema that resolve over hours. However, local reactions can be large (>4 cm in diameter), causing considerable discomfort and lasting more than 24 hours. These large local reactions may be associated with systemic reactions or be harbingers of a systemic reaction with higher doses of the immunotherapy. Immediate treatment of local reactions can be achieved through use of cold compresses or administration of an oral antihistamine or an injection of corticosteroid at the site. The dose of immunotherapy should be reduced when large local reactions occur.

Systemic reactions are a distinct risk for patients on immunotherapy. These may range from simple hives to severe life-threatening anaphylaxis. In some instances, systemic reactions have been fatal. Systemic reactions may be generalized urticaria and/or angioedema, swelling of the airway (tongue, throat, and lower airway) with impaired swallowing or breathing, or cold, damp skin, rapid pulse, and low blood pressure. In addition, there may be exacerbation of allergic symptoms such as sneezing, rhinorrhea, nasal congestion, wheezing, coughing, and shortness of breath. These must be differentiated from the vasovagal reactions of low blood pressure with low heart rate. The immediate treatment of systemic reactions is as follows:

1. Place the patient in a recumbent position
2. Inject aqueous epinephrine 1:1000 subcutaneously (0.3–0.5 ml for adults; 0.01 ml/kg body weight or 0.3 ml/m^2 for children)
3. Provide reassurance

Intravenous fluids may be given for the low blood pressure, oxygen for hypoxia, corticosteroid for prolonged reactions, CPR for cardiopulmonary arrest, and tracheal intubation for airway maintenance.

The American Academy of Allergy and Immunology has published recommended guidelines for practitioners giving immunotherapy. These are listed in Table 15-1. In addition, some physicians observe highly allergic individuals for 25 to 30 minutes after each injection. For asthmatic patients, immunotherapy should be administered only if the patient's peak flow or FEV$_1$ is greater than 75% of his or her personal best. In addition, immunotherapy probably should not be administered to patients on chronic β-

Table 15-1. Guidelines for Giving Immunotherapy

1. The patient should be observed for at least 20 minutes after the injection.
2. Office or clinic personnel should be familiar with:
   adjustment of the dose of allergenic extract to minimize reactions; recognition and treatment of local reactions; recognition and treatment of systemic reactions; and basic cardiopulmonary resuscitation.
3. Available equipment and reagents should include:
   stethoscope and sphygmomanometer, tourniquets, syringes, hypodermic needles, aqueous epinephrine HCl 1:1000, equipment for administration of oxygen by mask, oral airway, large bore needle (14 gauge) for tracheotomy, equipment for administering intravenous fluids, diphenhydramine or similar antihistamine, aminophylline for intravenous injection, corticosteroids for intravenous injection, and vasopressor.

blockers or having significant cardiovascular disease. In dealing with pregnant patients, immunotherapy should not be started, and for those patients already on immunotherapy but not on a maintenance dose, the current dose should be continued until the pregnancy is completed.

FUTURE OF IMMUNOTHERAPY

The future of immunotherapy is difficult to predict, but in the foreseeable future, the regimens and/or agents will be vastly different than they are today. Local nasal administration for immunotherapy has been tried and found to be effective in ragweed- and grass-sensitive patients. The advantages of such a program are that treatment can be given at home and is relatively safe and cost-effective. However, further studies are needed to elucidate the mechanism(s) of action and use of other aeroallergens. Recent work had implicated that anticytokine immunotherapy may be highly effective in altering the allergic response and is undergoing clinical trials.

SUMMARY

In summary, immunotherapy is not for every allergic patient, yet for those patients unresponsive to avoidance/environmental control and pharmacotherapeutic management, immunotherapy has been proven effective for allergic rhinitis and allergic asthma. Therapy, however, involves two to three years and has inherent risks of anaphylaxis and local reactions that the patient needs to be made aware of before instituting the injections.

SELECTED REFERENCES

Barnes PJ. Pathophysiology of allergic inflammation. In: Middleton EM Jr, Reed CE, Ellis EF, et al., eds. Allergy: principles and practice. St. Louis: C.V. Mosby, 1993:243–266.

Becker RJ. Whither allergy or wither allergy. Ann Allergy 1978;41:263–267.

Bruce CA, Norman PS, Rosenthal RR, Lichtenstein LM. The role of ragweed pollen in autumnal asthma. J Allergy Clin Immunol 1977;59:450.

Coca AF, Grove EF. Studies in hypersensitiveness. XIII. A study of the atopic reagins. J Immunol 1925;10:445–464.

Cooke RA, Barnard JH, Hebald S, Stull A. Serological evidence of immunity with coexisting sensitization in a type of allergy (hay fever). J Exp Med 1935;62:733–750.

Frankland AW, Augustin R. Prophylaxis of summer hayfever and asthma: a controlled trial comparing crude grass-pollen extracts with the isolated main protein component. Lancet 1954;1:1055–1057.

Freeman J. Further observations on the treatment of hay fever by hypodermic inoculations of pollen vaccine. Lancet 1911;2: 814–817.

Hagy GW, Settipane GA. Rhinitis. 2nd ed. Providence, RI: Oceanside Publishing, 1991.

Henderson WR Jr. The role of leukotrienes in inflammation. Ann Intern Med 1994;121:684–697.

Ishizaka K, Ishizaka T. Identification of IgE-antibodies as a carrier of reagenic activity. J Immunol 1967;99:1187–1197.

Lemanske RF, Kaliner MA. Late phase allergic reactions. In: Middleton EM Jr, Reed CE, Ellis EF, et al., eds. Allergy: principles and practice. St. Louis: C.V. Mosby, 1993:320–361.

Lowell FC, Franklin WA. A "double-blind" study of treatment with aqueous allergic extracts in cases of allergic rhinitis. J Allergy 1968;34:165–182.

Mayatepek E, Hoffman GF. Leukotrienes: biosynthesis, metabolism, and pathophysiologic significance. Pediatr Res 1995;37: 1–9.

McFadden ER Jr, Gilbert IA. Asthma. N Engl J Med 1992;327:1928–1937.

Naclerio RM. Allergic rhinitis. N Engl J Med 1991;325:860–869.

Noon L. Prophylactic inoculation against hay fever. Lancet 1911;1:1572–1573.

Norman PS. Safety of allergen immunotherapy. J Allergy Clin Immunol 1989;84:438–439.

Norman PS, Winkenwerder WL, Lichtenstein LM. Immunotherapy of hay fever with ragweed antigen E: comparisons with whole pollen extract and placebos. J Allergy 1968;42:93.

Ohman JL, Findlay SR, Leiterman M. Immunotherapy in cat-induced asthma. Double-blind trial with evaluation of in vivo and in vitro responses. J Allergy Clin Immunol 1984;74:230.

Ortolani C, Pastorello E, Moss RB, et al. Pollen immunotherapy: a single year double blind placebo-controlled study in patients with grass pollen induced asthma and rhinitis. J Allergy Clin Immunol 1984;73:284.

Parrish WE. Atopy: One hundred years of antibodies, mast cells and lymphocytes. Brit J Dermatol 1988;119:437–443.

Rocklin RE, Sheffer AL, Greineder DK, Melmon KL. Generation of antigen-specific suppressor cells during allergy desensitization. N Engl J Med 1980;302:1213–1219.

Settipane RJ, Hagy GW, Settipane GA. Long term risk factors for developing rhinitis: a 23 year follow-up study of college students. Allergy Proc 1994;15:21–25.

Taylor WW, Ohman JL, Lowell TC. Immunotherapy in cat-induced asthma. Double-blind trial with evaluation of bronchial responses to cat allergen and histamine. J Allergy Clin Immunol 1978;61:283.

Tinkelman DG, Cole WQ, Tunno J. Immunotherapy: a one-year prospective study to evaluate risk factors of systemic reactions. J Allergy Clin Immunol 1995;95:8–14.

Tuft L. Allergy practice during the early years. Ann Allergy 1982;49:238–243.

Unger L, Harris MC. Stepping stones in allergy. Chapter VII. The treatment of allergic diseases. Ann Allergy 1975;34:125–129.

Van Metre TE Jr, Adkinson NF Jr. Immunotherapy for aeroallergen disease. In: Middleton EM Jr, Reed CE, Ellis EF, et al., eds. Allergy: principles and practice. St. Louis: C.V. Mosby, 1993:1327–1343.

Weiss KB, Gergen PJ, Hodgson TA. An economic evaluation of asthma in the United States. N Engl J Med 1992;326:862–866.

Index

9671